17.95

W9-CBE-742

EXERCISE

GENERAL EDITORS

Dale C. Garell, M.D.
Medical Director, California Children Services, Department of Health
  Services, County of Los Angeles
Associate Dean for Curriculum; Clinical Professor, Department of Pediatrics &
  Family Medicine, University of Southern California School of Medicine
Former President, Society for Adolescent Medicine

Solomon H. Snyder, M.D.
Distinguished Service Professor of Neuroscience, Pharmacology, and
  Psychiatry, Johns Hopkins University School of Medicine
Former President, Society for Neuroscience
Albert Lasker Award in Medical Research, 1978

CONSULTING EDITORS

Robert W. Blum, M.D., Ph.D.
Associate Professor, School of Public Health and Department of
  Pediatrics
Director, Adolescent Health Program, University of Minnesota
  Consultant, World Health Organization

Charles E. Irwin, Jr., M.D.
Associate Professor of Pediatrics; Director, Division of Adolescent
  Medicine, University of California, San Francisco

Lloyd J. Kolbe, Ph.D.
Chief, Office of School Health & Special Projects, Center for Health
  Promotion & Education, Centers for Disease Control
President, American School Health Association

Jordan J. Popkin
Director, Division of Federal Employee Occupational Health, U.S. Public
  Health Service Region I

Joseph L. Rauh, M.D.
Professor of Pediatrics and Medicine, Adolescent Medicine, Children's
  Hospital Medical Center, Cincinnati
Former President, Society for Adolescent Medicine

Frank D. Rohter, Ph.D.
Professor, Department of Exceptional/Physical Education,
  University of Central Florida

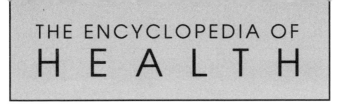

THE ENCYCLOPEDIA OF
HEALTH

THE HEALTHY BODY

Dale C. Garell, M.D. · General Editor

EXERCISE

Don Nardo

Introduction by C. Everett Koop, M.D., Sc.D.
former Surgeon General, U. S. Public Health Service

CHELSEA HOUSE PUBLISHERS

New York · Philadelphia

The goal of the ENCYCLOPEDIA OF HEALTH *is to provide general information in the ever-changing areas of physiology, psychology, and related medical issues. The titles in this series are not intended to take the place of the professional advice of a physician or other health care professional.*

ON THE COVER Computer-enhanced image of a man exercising

CHELSEA HOUSE PUBLISHERS
EDITOR-IN-CHIEF   Remmel Nunn
MANAGING EDITOR   Karyn Gullen Browne
COPY CHIEF   Mark Rifkin
PICTURE EDITOR   Adrian G. Allen
ART DIRECTOR   Maria Epes
ASSISTANT ART DIRECTOR   Noreen Romano
MANUFACTURING MANAGER   Gerald Levine
SYSTEMS MANAGER   Lindsey Ottman
PRODUCTION MANAGER   Joseph Romano
PRODUCTION COORDINATOR   Marie Claire Cebrián

The Encyclopedia of Health
SENIOR EDITOR   Brian Feinberg

Staff for EXERCISE
ASSOCIATE EDITOR   LaVonne Carlson-Finnerty
SENIOR COPY EDITOR   Laurie Kahn
EDITORIAL ASSISTANT   Tamar Levovitz
PICTURE RESEARCHER   Georganne Backman Garfinkel
DESIGNER   Robert Yaffe

First Printing
1   3   5   7   9   8   6   4   2

Library of Congress Cataloging-in-Publication Data

Nardo, Don.
  Exercise/by Don Nardo; introduction by C. Everett Koop.
    p.   cm.—(The Encyclopedia of health. The Healthy body)
  Includes bibliographical references and index.
  Summary: Examines exercise and its benefits and explores the subject of physical fitness.
  ISBN 0-7910-0017-6
      0-7910-0457-0 (pbk.)
  1. Exercise—Juvenile literature. 2. Physical fitness—Juvenile literature. [1. Exercise. 2. Physical fitness.] I. Title. II. Series: Encyclopedia of health. Healthy body.
                                                                              91-13308
GV481.N25 1991   CIP
613.7'1—dc20   AC

CONTENTS

"Prevention and Education:
The Keys to Good Health"—
C. Everett Koop, M.D., Sc.D.   7

Foreword—Dale C. Garell, M.D.   11

1   Physical Conditioning Through the Ages   13

2   The Muscles and How They Work   23

3   The Roles of the Heart and the Lungs   35

4   Exercise Types and Skills   49

5   The Importance of Nutrition   61

6   Behaviors That Impede Fitness   73

7   Creating a Personal Fitness Program   81

Appendix: For More Information   97

Further Reading   99

Glossary   104

Index   108

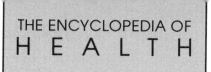

THE ENCYCLOPEDIA OF
H E A L T H

THE HEALTHY BODY

The Circulatory System
Dental Health
The Digestive System
The Endocrine System
Exercise
Genetics & Heredity
The Human Body: An Overview
Hygiene
The Immune System
Memory & Learning
The Musculoskeletal System
The Nervous System
Nutrition
The Reproductive System
The Respiratory System
The Senses
Sleep
Speech & Hearing
Sports Medicine
Vision
Vitamins & Minerals

THE LIFE CYCLE

Adolescence
Adulthood
Aging
Childhood
Death & Dying
The Family
Friendship & Love
Pregnancy & Birth

MEDICAL ISSUES

Careers in Health Care
Environmental Health
Folk Medicine
Health Care Delivery
Holistic Medicine
Medical Ethics
Medical Fakes & Frauds
Medical Technology
Medicine & the Law
Occupational Health
Public Health

PSYCHOLOGICAL DISORDERS AND THEIR TREATMENT

· Anxiety & Phobias
Child Abuse
Compulsive Behavior
Delinquency & Criminal Behavior
Depression
Diagnosing & Treating Mental Illness
Eating Habits & Disorders
Learning Disabilities
Mental Retardation
Personality Disorders
Schizophrenia
Stress Management
Suicide

MEDICAL DISORDERS AND THEIR TREATMENT

AIDS
Allergies
Alzheimer's Disease
Arthritis
Birth Defects
Cancer
The Common Cold
Diabetes
Emergency Medicine
Gynecological Disorders
Headaches
The Hospital
Kidney Disorders
Medical Diagnosis
The Mind-Body Connection
Mononucleosis and Other Infectious Diseases
Nuclear Medicine
Organ Transplants
Pain
Physical Handicaps
Poisons & Toxins
Prescription & OTC Drugs
Sexually Transmitted Diseases
Skin Disorders
Stroke & Heart Disease
Substance Abuse
Tropical Medicine

PREVENTION AND EDUCATION: THE KEYS TO GOOD HEALTH

C. Everett Koop, M.D., Sc.D.
former Surgeon General,
U.S. Public Health Service

The issue of health education has received particular attention in recent years because of the presence of AIDS in the news. But our response to this particular tragedy points up a number of broader issues that doctors, public health officials, educators, and the public face. In particular, it points up the necessity for sound health education for citizens of all ages.

Over the past 25 years this country has been able to bring about dramatic declines in the death rates for heart disease, stroke, accidents, and for people under the age of 45, cancer. Today, Americans generally eat better and take better care of themselves than ever before. Thus, with the help of modern science and technology, they have a better chance of surviving serious—even catastrophic—illnesses. That's the good news.

But, like every phonograph record, there's a flip side, and one with special significance for young adults. According to a report issued in 1979 by Dr. Julius Richmond, my predecessor as Surgeon General, Americans aged 15 to 24 had a higher death rate in 1979 than they did 20 years earlier. The causes: violent death and injury, alcohol and drug abuse, unwanted pregnancies, and sexually transmitted diseases. Adolescents are particularly vulnerable because they are beginning to explore their own sexuality and perhaps to experiment with drugs. The need for educating young people is critical, and the price of neglect is high.

Yet even for the population as a whole, our health is still far from what it could be. Why? A 1974 Canadian government report attributed all death and disease to four broad elements: inadequacies in the health care system, behavioral factors or unhealthy life-styles, environmental hazards, and human biological factors.

To be sure, there are diseases that are still beyond the control of even our advanced medical knowledge and techniques. And despite yearnings that are as old as the human race itself, there is no "fountain of youth" to ward off aging and death. Still, there is a solution to many of the problems that undermine sound health. In a word, that solution is prevention. Prevention, which includes health promotion and education, saves lives, improves the quality of life, and in the long run, saves money.

In the United States, organized public health activities and preventive medicine have a long history. Important milestones in this country or foreign breakthroughs adopted in the United States include the improvement of sanitary procedures and the development of pasteurized milk in the late 19th century and the introduction in the mid-20th century of effective vaccines against polio, measles, German measles, mumps, and other once-rampant diseases. Internationally, organized public health efforts began on a wide-scale basis with the International Sanitary Conference of 1851, to which 12 nations sent representatives. The World Health Organization, founded in 1948, continues these efforts under the aegis of the United Nations, with particular emphasis on combating communicable diseases and the training of health care workers.

Despite these accomplishments, much remains to be done in the field of prevention. For too long, we have had a medical care system that is science- and technology-based, focused, essentially, on illness and mortality. It is now patently obvious that both the social and the economic costs of such a system are becoming insupportable.

Implementing prevention—and its corollaries, health education and promotion—is the job of several groups of people.

First, the medical and scientific professions need to continue basic scientific research, and here we are making considerable progress. But increased concern with prevention will also have a decided impact on how primary care doctors practice medicine. With a shift to health-based rather than morbidity-based medicine, the role of the "new physician" will include a healthy dose of patient education.

Second, practitioners of the social and behavioral sciences—psychologists, economists, city planners—along with lawyers, business leaders, and government officials—must solve the practical and ethical dilemmas confronting us: poverty, crime, civil rights, literacy, education, employment, housing, sanitation, environmental protection, health care delivery systems, and so forth. All of these issues affect public health.

Third is the public at large. We'll consider that very important group in a moment.

Fourth, and the linchpin in this effort, is the public health profession—doctors, epidemiologists, teachers—who must harness the professional expertise of the first two groups and the common sense and cooperation of the third, the public. They must define the problems statistically and qualitatively and then help us set priorities for finding the solutions.

To a very large extent, improving those statistics is the responsibility of every individual. So let's consider more specifically what the role of the individual should be and why health education is so important to that role. First, and most obvious, individuals can protect themselves from illness and injury and thus minimize their need for professional medical care. They can eat nutritious food; get adequate exercise; avoid tobacco, alcohol, and drugs; and take prudent steps to avoid accidents. The proverbial "apple a day keeps the doctor away" is not so far from the truth, after all.

Second, individuals should actively participate in their own medical care. They should schedule regular medical and dental checkups. Should they develop an illness or injury, they should know when to treat themselves and when to seek professional help. To gain the maximum benefit from any medical treatment that they do require, individuals must become partners in that treatment. For instance, they should understand the effects and side effects of medications. I counsel young physicians that there is no such thing as too much information when talking with patients. But the corollary is the patient must know enough about the nuts and bolts of the healing process to understand what the doctor is telling him or her. That is at least partially the patient's responsibility.

Education is equally necessary for us to understand the ethical and public policy issues in health care today. Sometimes individuals will encounter these issues in making decisions about their own treatment or that of family members. Other citizens may encounter them as jurors in medical malpractice cases. But we all become involved, indirectly, when we elect our public officials, from school board members to the president. Should surrogate parenting be legal? To what extent is drug testing desirable, legal, or necessary? Should there be public funding for family planning, hospitals, various types of medical research, and other medical care for the indigent? How should we allocate scant technological resources, such as kidney dialysis and organ transplants? What is the proper role of government in protecting the rights of patients?

What are the broad goals of public health in the United States today? In 1980, the Public Health Service issued a report aptly entitled *Promoting Health—Preventing Disease: Objectives for the Nation*. This report expressed its goals in terms of mortality and in terms of intermediate goals in education and health improvement. It identified 15 major concerns: controlling high blood pressure; improving family planning; improving pregnancy care and infant health; increasing the rate of immunization; controlling sexually transmitted diseases; controlling the presence of toxic agents and radiation in the environment; improving occupational safety and health; preventing accidents; promoting water fluoridation and dental health; controlling infectious diseases; decreasing smoking; decreasing alcohol and drug abuse; improving nutrition; promoting physical fitness and exercise; and controlling stress and violent behavior.

For healthy adolescents and young adults (ages 15 to 24), the specific goal was a 20% reduction in deaths, with a special focus on motor vehicle injuries and alcohol and drug abuse. For adults (ages 25 to 64), the aim was 25% fewer deaths, with a concentration on heart attacks, strokes, and cancers.

Smoking is perhaps the best example of how individual behavior can have a direct impact on health. Today, cigarette smoking is recognized as the single most important preventable cause of death in our society. It is responsible for more cancers and more cancer deaths than any other known agent; is a prime risk factor for heart and blood vessel disease, chronic bronchitis, and emphysema; and is a frequent cause of complications in pregnancies and of babies born prematurely, underweight, or with potentially fatal respiratory and cardiovascular problems.

Since the release of the Surgeon General's first report on smoking in 1964, the proportion of adult smokers has declined substantially, from 43% in 1965 to 30.5% in 1985. Since 1965, 37 million people have quit smoking. Although there is still much work to be done if we are to become a "smoke-free society," it is heartening to note that public health and public education efforts—such as warnings on cigarette packages and bans on broadcast advertising—have already had significant effects.

In 1835, Alexis de Tocqueville, a French visitor to America, wrote, "In America the passion for physical well-being is general." Today, as then, health and fitness are front-page items. But with the greater scientific and technological resources now available to us, we are in a far stronger position to make good health care available to everyone. And with the greater technological threats to us as we approach the 21st century, the need to do so is more urgent than ever before. Comprehensive information about basic biology, preventive medicine, medical and surgical treatments, and related ethical and public policy issues can help you arm yourself with the knowledge you need to be healthy throughout your life.

FOREWORD

Dale C. Garell, M.D.

Advances in our understanding of health and disease during the 20th century have been truly remarkable. Indeed, it could be argued that modern health care is one of the greatest accomplishments in all of human history. In the early 20th century, improvements in sanitation, water treatment, and sewage disposal reduced death rates and increased longevity. Previously untreatable illnesses can now be managed with antibiotics, immunizations, and modern surgical techniques. Discoveries in the fields of immunology, genetic diagnosis, and organ transplantation are revolutionizing the prevention and treatment of disease. Modern medicine is even making inroads against cancer and heart disease, two of the leading causes of death in the United States.

Although there is much to be proud of, medicine continues to face enormous challenges. Science has vanquished diseases such as smallpox and polio, but new killers, most notably AIDS, confront us. Moreover, we now victimize ourselves with what some have called "diseases of choice," or those brought on by drug and alcohol abuse, bad eating habits, and mismanagement of the stresses and strains of contemporary life. The very technology that is doing so much to prolong life has brought with it previously unimaginable ethical dilemmas related to issues of death and dying. The rising cost of health care is a matter of central concern to us all. And violence in the form of automobile accidents, homicide, and suicide remains the major killer of young adults.

In the past, most people were content to leave health care and medical treatment in the hands of professionals. But since the 1960s, the consumer of medical care—that is, the patient—has assumed an increasingly central role in the management of his or her own health. There has also been a new emphasis placed on prevention: People are recognizing that their own actions can help prevent many of the conditions that have caused death and disease in the past. This accounts for the growing commitment to good nutrition and regular exercise, for the increasing number of people who are choosing not to smoke, and for a new moderation in people's drinking habits.

People want to know more about themselves and their own health. They are curious about their body: its anatomy, physiology, and biochemistry. They want to keep up with rapidly evolving medical technologies and procedures. They are willing to educate themselves about common disorders and diseases so that they can be full partners in their own health care.

THE ENCYCLOPEDIA OF HEALTH is designed to provide the basic knowledge that readers will need if they are to take significant responsibility for their own health. It is also meant to serve as a frame of reference for further study and exploration. The encyclopedia is divided into five subsections: The Healthy Body; The Life Cycle; Medical Disorders & Their Treatment; Psychological Disorders & Their Treatment; and Medical Issues. For each topic covered by the encyclopedia, we present the essential facts about the relevant biology; the symptoms, diagnosis, and treatment of common diseases and disorders; and ways in which you can prevent or reduce the severity of health problems when that is possible. The encyclopedia also projects what may lie ahead in the way of future treatment or prevention strategies.

The broad range of topics and issues covered in the encyclopedia reflects that human health encompasses physical, psychological, social, environmental, and spiritual well-being. Just as the mind and the body are inextricably linked, so, too, is the individual an integral part of the wider world that comprises his or her family, society, and environment. To discuss health in its broadest aspect it is necessary to explore the many ways in which it is connected to such fields as law, social science, public policy, economics, and even religion. And so, the encyclopedia is meant to be a bridge between science, medical technology, the world at large, and you. I hope that it will inspire you to pursue in greater depth particular areas of interest and that you will take advantage of the suggestions for further reading and the lists of resources and organizations that can provide additional information.

CHAPTER 1

PHYSICAL CONDITIONING THROUGH THE AGES

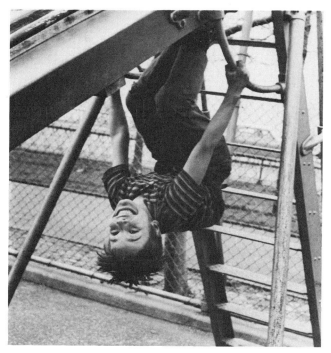

For children, play is a fun way to condition a growing body.

As the medical community gains increasing knowledge about the harmful, sometimes crippling effects of a sedentary life-style, more and more people are making exercise an important part of their day. Yet even now, many other individuals remain weak, couch-bound, and overweight.

DEVICE FOR DEVELOPMENT

Youngsters first begin exercising when they play—a painless way of conditioning their growing body. Typical children are full of energy and are constantly running, jumping, and climbing. Play not only keeps the muscles and heart fit but also develops coordination, flexibility, and other abilities. "The young child perhaps learns more and develops better through his play than through any other form of activity," suggested American educator Herbert S. Jennings (1868–1947).

Unfortunately, the majority of American children become increasingly inactive as they get older. Studies have shown that by age 15 or 16, most get little or no regular exercise outside of school gym classes, and many children end up overweight and out of shape. Educators first noticed this trend during the 1960s. Although schools have increased their emphasis on teaching the values of exercise and fitness since that time, the problem has not gone away.

Indeed, those who are inactive as teenagers tend not to improve their habits later in life. Because of continued lack of regular exercise and poor diet, many American adults are overweight and suffer from health problems ranging from shortness of breath and backaches to depression and heart disease. Destructive habits such as smoking, alcohol consumption, and drug abuse also remain common and can cause further damage to health.

EXERCISE THROUGH HISTORY

Lack of activity destroys the good condition of every human being, while movement and methodical physical exercise save it and preserve it.

— Plato (350 B.C.)

The knowledge that regular exercise keeps the body fit is not a recent discovery. People have been exercising for thousands of years, although each culture had its own reasons for staying in shape.

Warding Off the Ills of Inactivity

More than 40 centuries ago, the Chinese recognized that individuals who exercised several times a week got sick less frequently than inactive people did. In fact, the Chinese believed that many diseases were actually caused by inactivity. So in 2689 B.C., the Chinese developed *kong fu,* a set of gymnastic exercises designed to promote fitness as well as personal discipline. Some of these exercises were related to self-defense and, over the centuries, they evolved into the modern version of the regimen, called *kung fu.*

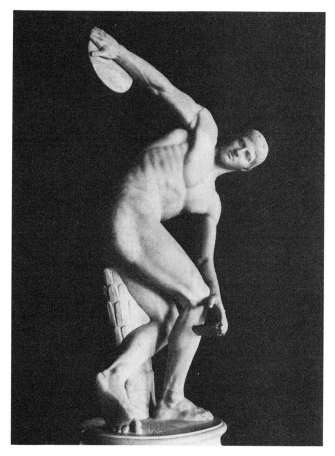

A discus thrower from ancient Greece; almost 2,500 years ago, the Greeks considered it important to develop both the body and the mind, in order to produce a well-rounded individual.

But in ancient India, the Hindu and Buddhist religions stressed the virtues of quiet, spiritual pursuits. The priests frowned upon games, sports, and exercise, claiming that these things satisfied the body rather than the spirit. However, it appears that only the most devout Indians actually adhered to the religious prohibitions against exercise, and such activities as chariot racing, horseback riding, wrestling, boxing, and dancing were popular. The most disciplined individuals studied Hindu *yoga,* a series of 84 exercises stressing flexibility, regulated breathing, and deep concentration. Eventually, the priests adopted yoga and used it as a means of clearing the mind for prayer. Yoga is still practiced today in India and in many other parts of the world.

Training for War

For the ancient Egyptians, exercise played a decidedly different role. It was used mainly as a means of preparing strong bodies for battle. Physical fitness was practiced almost solely by males with the primary goal of building stronger, more effective armies. Young Egyptian boys were trained in the use of the bow and arrow, battle-ax, lance, and other weapons. They also performed exercises that increased their endurance, such as running, marching, and wrestling.

Like the Egyptians, the ancient Persians saw exercise as a way to prepare young men for warfare. But the Persians, whose military traditions were unusually aggressive, took the idea of physical conditioning to a greater extreme. At the time that the Persian Empire reached its greatest size and influence (about 530 B.C.), it was customary for all young boys to begin their military training at age six. Soldiers removed the boys from their homes and subjected them to vigorous, often harsh physical fitness routines; they also instructed the boys in both the bow and arrow and the javelin, as well as in riding and marching. To prepare the children for the hardships of war, the soldiers often starved the boys and forced them to exercise for hours in extremes of heat and cold. No effort was given to training the boys' minds, since the intellectual development of the individual was considered useless to the state. The only activities stressed were those that strengthened the army's ability to conquer and destroy.

The Well-Rounded Individual

In sharp contrast to the military-oriented approach to exercise of the Egyptians and Persians, the Greeks saw physical conditioning as a way to help them become better people. Although this quest for self-betterment became a common feature of life in many of the Greek city-states, it was most characteristic of the inhabitants of Athens, the birthplace of democracy. During the classical, or "golden age" of Athens (about 500–350 B.C.), a unique vision of the human being developed. It stressed the importance of the whole, or well-rounded, individual, striving for excellence in both physical and mental pursuits. To the Greeks, exercise and learning went hand in hand.

The Greeks were the first people in history to emphasize the artistic beauty of the human body. For them, the primary goal of exercise was to achieve a state of physical excellence. They performed gymnastic exercises of all types, believing these helped build a whole person. The exercises not only developed strength and courage and promoted good

The first Olympic Games were held in Greece in 776 B.C. Winners, rewarded with a wreath of olive branches, were considered national heroes.

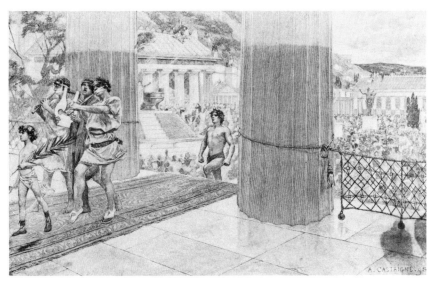

health but also taught the participants the importance of fair play. The Greeks championed the idea of amateurism in sports and banned professional competitions, which offered material rewards to the winners. The rewards for physical fitness, the Greeks believed, should be personal—the attainment of good health and a beautiful body.

The Greek quest for physical excellence reached its highest expression in the *Olympic Games,* first held in the Greek town of Olympia in 776 B.C. There, athletes ran, threw the discus and javelin, boxed, wrestled, and raced horses before a crowd of more than 40,000 spectators. The winner of each event received only a wreath of olive branches but was looked upon as a national hero. Participants competed in the nude in order to emphasize the glory of the well-conditioned human body.

Stressing the Practical and the Cruel

The Romans, like the Greeks, saw exercise as a means of achieving better health. Unlike the Greeks, however, the Romans stressed physical fitness more for its value in building stronger soldiers and laborers. Thus, to the Romans, a conservative and very practical people, physical attributes such as strength and endurance were best used to serve the needs and desires of the empire, not the individual. The Romans rejected the Greek idea of exercising to achieve a beautiful body and found the sight of nude athletes embarrassing. The Romans also preferred professionalism to amateurism and liked gory, often cruel, spectator sports such as gladiator fights and battles to the death between men and animals.

After the fall of Rome in the fifth century A.D., Christianity quickly spread across Europe. In the following centuries, referred to as the Middle Ages, the Church frowned upon physical conditioning, emphasizing instead more scholarly pursuits. There were no gymnastic competitions or spectator sports, and even military organizations did not emphasize formal physical training as much as the Romans had. In time, few people paid any attention to the idea of exercise and physical fitness.

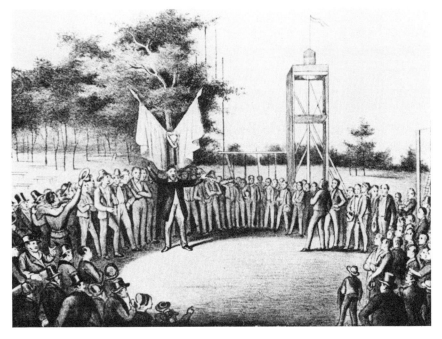

During the 19th century, German educator Friedrich Ludwig Jahn helped create a new respect for fitness and exercise. Seen here speaking to a crowd of enthusiasts, he created a program of exercises for students that included jumping, vaulting, climbing, balancing, and running.

This situation began to change in the late Middle Ages, when feudal lords started maintaining garrisons and even small armies of armored knights. The knights underwent a rigorous training regimen. Exercise and physical fitness were used to prepare not only for combat but also for increasingly popular competitive sports such as jousting and fencing.

The Spread of Physical Education

Modern ideas about exercise and fitness began developing in the 18th century, mainly in Germany, Denmark, and Britain. Social leaders and educators of the time argued that any country that promoted regular exercise for most of its citizens would become militarily stronger. At the same time, it would have a healthier, more productive populace. Exercise advocates such as Johann Basedow (1723–90), Johann Christoph Muths (1759–1839), and Adolph Spiess (1810–58) maintained that the best way to promote physical fitness was to institute sports and exercise programs in the schools.

Particularly influential in spreading the idea of a fit society was the German educator Friedrich Ludwig Jahn (1778–1852), who set up a program of exercises for students. This included jumping, vaulting, climbing, balancing, and running. He also invented and built various types of gymnastic equipment to aid the students in their training. Jahn's system quickly became popular, and clubs, or "societies," that stressed his methods sprang up all over Germany and in other parts of Europe. In 1870, there were 1,500 such organizations. By 1890, there were 4,000 Jahn societies, and by 1920, more than 10,000 around the world.

Exercise in the United States

The idea of regular exercise gained favor very slowly in America, and during the colonial period there was very little stress on such activities. By the late 18th and early 19th centuries, however, some of the fitness concepts popular in Europe had begun to take hold in the United States. A few American schools and academies introduced regular exercise,

A women's gymnastics class, New York, early 20th century; during the 1820s, Jahn's training programs were introduced in the United States, and by 1900, most American schools had adopted physical education.

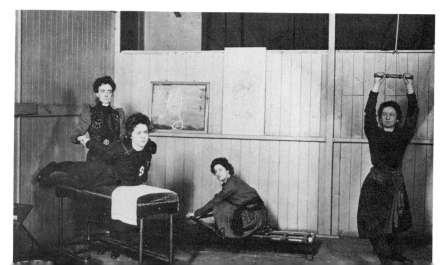

games, and sports as a means of keeping students healthy so they would miss less school due to illness. These activities also proved valuable in relieving the often monotonous routine of classes and studies.

During the 1820s, educators Charles Beck and Charles Follen introduced Jahn's gymnastic training programs to schools in Massachusetts. Later, more German exercise programs were instituted in St. Louis and other midwestern cities. By 1900, most American schools had adopted physical education programs that emphasized the importance of regular exercise.

Another factor that encouraged the idea of exercise in America was the rise of popular sports. In the late 19th century, activities such as tennis, golf, wrestling, boxing, track, squash, swimming, and skiing gained large followings in the United States. During this same period, Americans invented some popular sports of their own, including basketball. Organized baseball, which originated in Hoboken, New Jersey, had been around since about 1846.

In the 20th century, many sports, including baseball, became huge American institutions, drawing large crowds to both indoor and outdoor stadiums. At the same time, high schools and colleges organized formal sports programs. Exercise programs, however, remained oriented mostly to school and professional sports until the 1970s. It then became increasingly popular for individuals outside of formal sports to practice their own regular fitness programs. For instance, jogging became a popular pastime, and health clubs and spas, once few in number, multiplied all over the country. In addition, *aerobics* classes

Baseball game, 1887; the rise of popular sports helped encourage exercise in America.

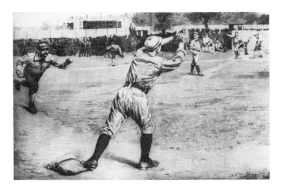

(see Chapter 4) gained a wide following in the 1970s and 1980s. Dr. Frank D. Rohter, an exercise physiologist and a professor at the University of Central Florida, has described several reasons behind the popularity of aerobic exercise, pointing out that jogging (an aerobic activity) found favor because it is simple to do and requires little in the way of equipment.

Today, a great many Americans recognize the importance of physical fitness and know that regular exercise can help them maintain better health and live longer. Although large numbers of people remain inactive, many individuals sincerely want to get into shape, and joggers have become an increasingly common sight. Most of those who manage to stay on their exercise routines and get into shape have some of the same goals as the ancients. Like the Chinese, they know that inactivity leads to illness, and so they exercise for good health. Some follow the example of the Greeks and seek to improve their physique. Others, like the first practitioners of yoga, find that exercise clears their mind, relaxes them, and puts them more in touch with themselves. Whatever their personal goals, exercise advocates seem to have something in common—most say they do it because they enjoy it.

CHAPTER 2

THE MUSCLES AND HOW THEY WORK

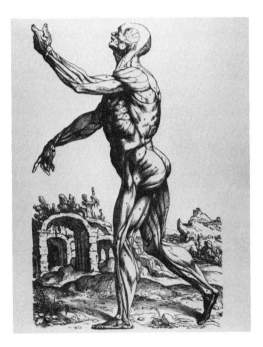

Muscles move the body, pump the blood, and pull air into the lungs. (The *diaphragm,* which controls breathing, is a wall of muscle.) An understanding of how the muscles work is important to any examination of exercise.

MUSCLE TISSUE

Most muscles in the human body are called *skeletal muscles* because they are attached to the bones, which make up the skeleton, by pieces of tough white tissue called *tendons.* Skeletal muscles make up about 40% of the total body weight of an average person.

The tissue of each muscle is composed of individual cells called *fibers.* Most cells in the body, blood cells for example, are very tiny and about as wide as they are long. By contrast, muscle fibers are relatively long and large. The fibers in a muscle are not evenly spaced but are bound together in tight bundles. There are about 100 to 150 separate fibers in each bundle and several bundles in each muscle. Usually, the larger the muscle, the more bundles it contains. The fibers and bundles are held together by strong groups of cells known as connective tissue.

Muscle tissue is elastic, which means that it stretches and bends rather easily. This elastic quality not only makes individual movements easier but also allows the length of a muscle to be changed through exercise. For instance, a muscle that is constantly stretched will eventually become a bit longer and allow for more flexible movements. On the other hand, a muscle that is constantly tightened will eventually get shorter, thicker, and stronger.

The skeletal muscles are almost always in a low state of tension, or firmness. This firm quality is called *tonus,* more commonly referred to as *muscle tone.* Muscle tone is involuntary, which means that a person does not have to think about flexing his or her muscles in order to keep them toned. Instead, the brain constantly sends signals to the muscle fibers, ordering them to maintain tone and giving them the amount of tension they need to maintain the body's normal posture. Without normal muscle tone, people would not be able to remain standing or even to hold up their head without making a conscious effort.

THE IMPORTANCE OF MUSCLE USE

In order to maintain their tone, muscles require constant use. In a sense, then, everyday activities such as sitting up, bending over, walking,

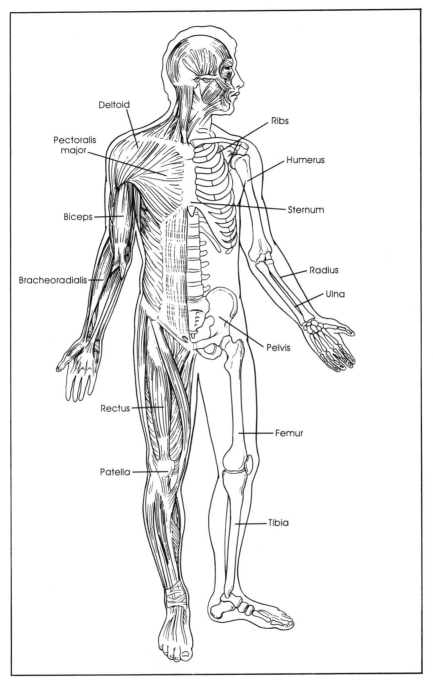

Diagram of the musculoskeletal system; most of the body's muscles are skeletal muscles, which means they are attached to bones. Muscle contractions make movement possible.

cooking, and writing are mild forms of exercise. Lack of use causes muscles to deteriorate and lose some of their strength and tone, a condition known as *atrophy.* The less active a person is, the more his or her muscles will atrophy.

In most cases, atrophy is mild and can be overcome by increased activity. Occasionally, however, a muscle or group of muscles is not used at all and becomes extremely deteriorated. For example, when a broken leg remains immobilized in a cast for many weeks, the leg muscles are severely weakened. One, two, or more weeks of special exercises may be needed to return the muscles to their normal strength after the break has healed.

MUSCLE CONTRACTIONS

In order to put the body in motion, muscles must *contract.* Most of the time, a contracting muscle gets shorter and thicker. For instance, the muscle in the front of the upper arm, the *bicep,* becomes rounder and more compact when the arm is flexed. Sometimes, a contracting muscle gets longer, as is the case when a person bends over. The muscles in

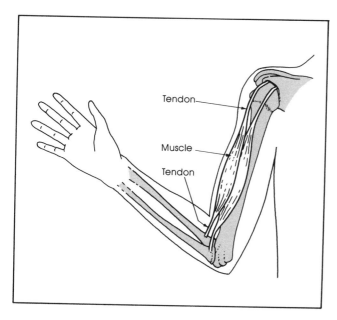

Skeletal muscles are attached to bones by pieces of tough white tissue called tendons.

the lower and middle back stretch and tighten in an effort to overcome the pull of gravity and hold up the upper body.

There are two general types of muscle contractions. The first, an *isotonic contraction,* is one that results in some kind of movement. For example, when a person contracts a bicep, the forearm moves upward toward the contracting muscle. Whenever someone lifts, pulls, or pushes on an object, forcing the object to move, the person's muscles have experienced isotonic contractions.

The second type of muscle contraction is an *isometric contraction,* in which the muscle tightens but nothing moves. A common example is that of someone trying to move an object that is much too heavy. As the person strains to lift, the muscles contract tightly, but the object does not budge. The individual's arms, back, and other body parts involved in the lifting effort do not move, either. Whenever someone lifts, pulls, or pushes an object but fails to move it, the person's muscles have experienced isometric contractions.

Muscle tissue is composed of individual cells called fibers. Skeletal muscle tissue is striated (lined) and its contractions are under the brain's conscious control. Cardiac (heart) muscle is also striated, but smooth muscle is not. Movement of both cardiac and smooth muscle (such as the pumping of the heart) is automatic, requiring no conscious thought.

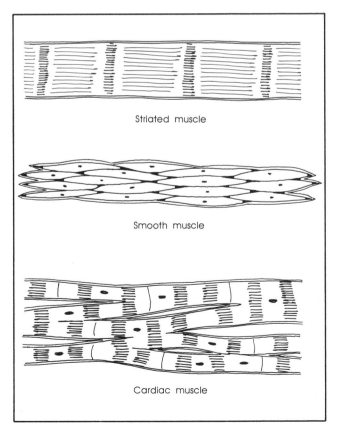

Striated muscle

Smooth muscle

Cardiac muscle

BODYBUILDING: RECAPTURING THE GREEK IDEAL

The modern sport of bodybuilding has developed only within the past 100 years. Prior to that, wrestlers and circus strongmen had been interested mainly in increasing their strength. The early bodybuilders, however, wanted to develop a physique that was well proportioned and pleasing to look at, resurrecting the ancient Greek ideal that stressed the artistic beauty of the human body.

The first person in modern times to gain a widespread reputation for his physique was Eugene Sandow, who traveled to America from Europe in the 1890s. Through years of lifting barbells and dumbbells, he greatly increased the size and definition of his muscles. Billed as the World's Strongest Man, he toured the United States performing feats of strength. Unlike traditional circus strongmen, however, Sandow also did something new: Wearing only a fig leaf, he would stand in a glass case and pose, allowing the audience to marvel at his unusual muscular development.

Thanks to Sandow, lifting weights quickly gained in popularity. In 1903, publisher Bermarr Macfadden ran the first Most Perfectly Developed Man in America contest in New York City. The idea caught on and the competition became an annual event. The 1921 winner, Angelo Siciliano, changed his name to Charles Atlas and began to advertise fitness programs in the back of magazines and comic books. That is how many young boys from the 1920s through the 1970s first became aware of bodybuilding.

In 1939, the Amateur Athletic Union began its now famous Mr. America contest to determine who had the most impressive physique. The Mr. Universe competition was introduced shortly afterward, and the first bodybuilder to win both titles was Steve Reeves, who later portrayed Hercules in several low-budget films of the 1950s.

Many young bodybuilders of the 1960s tried to emulate Reeves as well as other well-known competitors, such as Reg Park, Frank Zane, and Bill Pearl. New contests were introduced, such as the Mr. World and Mr. Olympia competitions. In addition, some women now began to lift weights and compete as bodybuilders.

Yet most of the general public still considered bodybuilding an odd, fringe sport and regarded bodybuilders themselves as muscle-bound and obsessed with their body.

This attitude changed in the 1970s with the appearance of both the book and the movie versions of *Pumping Iron.* The documentary gave the public insight into the sport of bodybuilding by portraying the training, goals, and everyday life of its competitors. The sport suddenly gained in popularity and respectability, earning coverage in network sports broadcasts and major magazines. *Pumping Iron* also launched the international career of its principal subject, champion bodybuilder Arnold Schwarzenegger, who went on to become a top movie star.

Champion bodybuilders are extremely dedicated and disciplined athletes. They must spend long hours in the gym several times a week for years to achieve their impressive physique. However, some bodybuilders have also been known to put themselves on extreme diets that include severe and unhealthy restrictions on fat intake. Steroid use has also been a problem among the bodybuilding community. Nonetheless, athletes can pursue the sport without such damaging shortcuts.

Bodybuilders believe that training does more than just enlarge their muscles; they claim that the sport contributes positively to every other aspect of their life. Schwarzenegger, in his book *Encyclopedia of Modern Bodybuilding,* insisted, "Bodybuilding means so much more today than it did when I first fell in love with it. Then, there was only competition, but now it has developed a recreational side—bodybuilding for fitness, health, and developing confidence and a better self-image."

The public's perception of bodybuilding has evolved over the decades, so that what was once considered a fringe sport is now an accepted part of athletics.

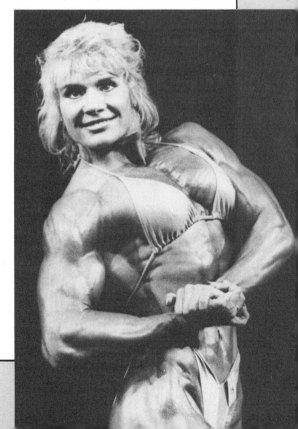

MUSCLE EFFICIENCY

Certain factors influence the ability of the muscles to contract, whether they are used to accomplish simple, everyday tasks or to perform strenuous, repeated exercises. One of these factors is the *warm-up*. The performance of a muscle is improved if the muscle is slightly warmed up by a period of moderate exercise before it undergoes a major contraction. This is one reason sprinters do warm-up exercises before a race. The exercises warm up the leg muscles so that they will contract more efficiently during the sprint. Another example is that of baseball pitchers, who often pitch better on warm days. If a muscle that is not warmed up suddenly undergoes a violent contraction, the muscle can stretch too far or even tear.

Another factor that affects the performance of the muscles is *fatigue*. When a muscle becomes fatigued from repeated use, its ability to contract and accomplish work is decreased. For instance, the longer a person swims, the harder it becomes to continue stroking with the arms and shoulders. Eventually, the muscles feel weak and begin to ache, and the person must rest.

Muscle fatigue is caused by the buildup of *lactic acid* in the muscle tissues. Lactic acid is a waste product of the substance *glycogen,* which the muscles burn for fuel. When muscles do not receive enough oxygen during the glycogen conversion process, lactic acid forms; the more lactic acid produced, the less efficiently the muscle performs.

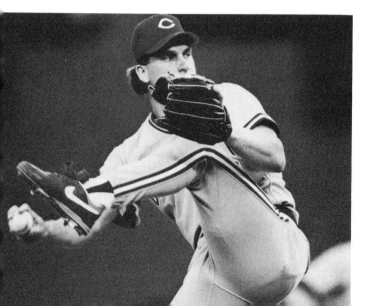

Muscles perform better at higher temperatures. This is why baseball pitchers, such as Rob Dibble of the Cincinnati Reds, need to warm-up before taking the mound and why baseball players prefer not to play in cold weather.

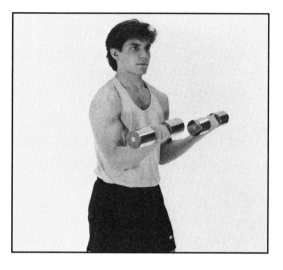

Some athletes prefer to train their muscles primarily for strength by lifting extremely heavy weights just a few times per workout. Others, however, strive for muscular endurance by using lighter weights to perform more repetitions.

STRENGTH AND ENDURANCE

Strength and *endurance* are measures of the amount of work a muscle or muscle group can perform. Strength is usually defined as the amount of force that can be applied by one or more muscles in a single contraction. Consider someone using one arm to lift a dumbbell. The individual puts as much effort as possible into the action and manages to lift the dumbbell once. The person's strength can be determined by the weight of the dumbbell. Obviously, someone who can lift a 100-pound dumbbell is a good deal stronger than someone else who can lift at most a 30-pound dumbbell.

Muscular endurance is the ability of a muscle to contract repeatedly. For instance, a person who can lift a 20-pound dumbbell 40 times in a row has more muscular endurance than someone who can lift the same dumbbell 30 times.

Strength and endurance are related. Usually, as a muscle's strength increases, so does its endurance. However, the two factors do not necessarily increase proportionally. Suppose that the person who lifted the 100-pound dumbbell once can lift the 20-pound dumbbell 50 times in succession. It does not automatically follow that another individual who is unable to lift the 100-pound dumbbell once has less endurance than the first person. The second person, though not as strong as the first, might be capable of lifting the 20-pound weight 60 times, exhibiting greater muscular endurance.

A comparison of Olympic weight lifters and swimmers clearly illustrates this point. The weight lifters have more sheer strength, having trained their muscles to expend a tremendous amount of energy in one or two major contractions. By contrast, the swimmers, though not as strong, can produce many more smaller contractions over a longer period of time than the weight lifters can. Thus, the swimmers have more endurance.

When inactive muscles atrophy, both strength and endurance are reduced. That is why athletes who stop competing and training get out of shape. In addition, as people age, they often tend to be less active and so have less strength and endurance. It should be noted that inactivity affects endurance more than strength. For instance, some people in their seventies still retain a great degree of muscular strength but tire easily because of loss of endurance.

HOW EXERCISE MAKES MUSCLES GROW

Both physique and body composition can be altered through exercise. The term *muscular physique* describes the sizes and proportions of the various muscles and muscle groups. Repeated strenuous exercise over a period of months or years can slowly increase the size of specific muscles. At the same time, exercise can define, or sharpen, the shape of the muscles.

To produce noticeable muscle growth, a person must regularly *overload* the muscles—that is, exercise very vigorously.

During each such exercise session, cells in the muscle tissue experience severe fatigue. Many of the cells become temporarily unable to function normally. During a rest period of hours or days, the muscle cells recover, after which the muscle tissue is a bit harder and stronger than it was before exercising. Certain exercises, especially those in which the muscles must contract to lift heavy weights, can slowly increase the size of the muscles.

Thus, over the course of time, a person can change his or her muscular physique through exercise, as clearly evidenced by competitive bodybuilders like Arnold Schwarzenegger. The muscle-building process can be quite selective. A person who wants to increase a

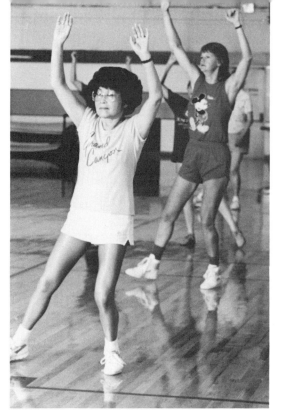

As people age, they often become less active, and their muscles lose strength and endurance. Exercise, even among senior citizens, can combat the problem.

muscle's size will concentrate on exercises that emphasize muscular strength, causing the muscle to contract with maximum force only a few times. On the other hand, a person who wants to sharpen a muscle's shape and definition will perform exercises that emphasize muscular endurance. This individual will make the muscle contract with a minimal amount of force many times in succession.

Often, a certain type of muscle development automatically comes with playing a specific sport. Long-distance runners, who train for endurance, have lean, sharply defined leg muscles. By contrast, wrestlers must sometimes bridge up on their neck in order to keep their shoulders off the mat, forcing their neck muscles to hold up their entire body weight for short periods. This action increases the strength of the muscles and often causes the wrestlers' neck to become noticeably thicker. And, as mentioned earlier, bodybuilders compete by specifically altering various muscles and muscle groups to achieve a completely new physique.

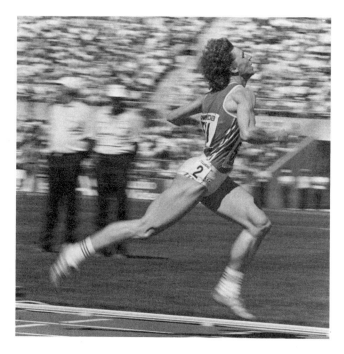

Specific sports often lead to a specific type of muscle development. For example, long-distance runners, trained for physical endurance, are known for having lean, well-defined leg muscles.

The term *body composition* usually refers to the proportions of muscle and fat in a person's arms, legs, chest, and other areas of the body. Regular exercise tends to alter body composition by increasing the ratio of muscle to fat. Usually, when a person exercises strenuously and often, the amount of fat surrounding the muscles decreases. Thus, by eliminating excess fat, exercise can give a person a leaner physique. Unfortunately, this effect is not permanent. To maintain it, the person must continue exercising, since fat deposits tend to build up again during periods of inactivity.

Exercise is essential to keeping muscles fit. The human muscular system is very much like a machine in that it allows people to accomplish work. Moreover, like the parts of a complicated machine, the muscles of the body need to be properly maintained to assure maximum efficiency. This means they must be exercised regularly.

CHAPTER 3

THE ROLES OF THE HEART AND THE LUNGS

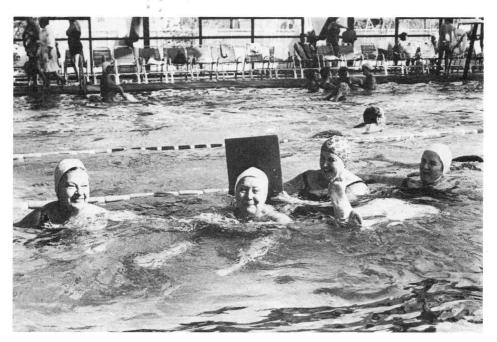

Regular exercise increases both cardiovascular and respiratory endurance and can keep the body working efficiently well into old age.

The body tissues, including the muscles, require a constant supply of oxygen in order to keep working efficiently. The *cardiovascular* and *respiratory* systems function together to supply the tissues with the oxygen they need.

The oxygen requirements of the muscle tissues are highest during exercise. When the body is at rest, the muscles consume about 20% of the oxygen provided by the cardiovascular and respiratory systems. This consumption increases dramatically when a person begins to work out. During vigorous activity, the muscles need up to 50 times the amount of oxygen they require when they are at rest.

EXERCISE AND THE HEART

The cardiovascular system is designed to carry food and oxygen to the body's tissue cells and also to ferry away the wastes that cells produce. The three basic components of the system are the blood, the blood vessels, and the heart.

The heart is a muscular organ about the size of a fist. Its job is to pump blood containing nutrients and oxygen to various parts of the body. The heart is made up of four hollow chambers. The muscular walls of these chambers contract in a regular pattern, squeezing blood with great force from the upper chambers into the lower ones, and from the lower chambers into the blood vessels.

The amount, or volume, of blood the heart pumps from the left or right ventricle per minute is called its *cardiac output*. When a person

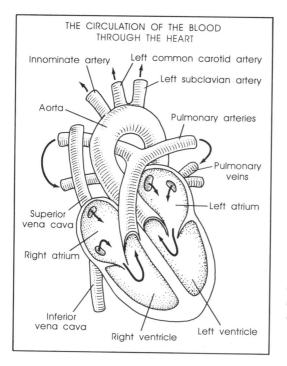

THE CIRCULATION OF THE BLOOD
THROUGH THE HEART

Innominate artery — Left common carotid artery — Left subclavian artery — Aorta — Pulmonary arteries — Pulmonary veins — Left atrium — Superior vena cava — Right atrium — Inferior vena cava — Right ventricle — Left ventricle

Blood enters the right side of the heart through the two venae cavae, flows from the right atrium into the right ventricle, and is pumped out through the pulmonary trunk to pick up oxygen from the lungs. Then the blood circulates back toward the heart, entering the left atrium through the pulmonary veins and flowing into the left ventricle. From there it is pumped through the aorta and into the arteries to bring oxygen to the rest of the body.

is at rest, the body tissues need only minimal amounts of oxygen and nutrients, so cardiac output is also minimal. The average heart pumps more than five quarts of blood per minute when the person is at rest; this is referred to as the normal *resting value* of cardiac output.

When a person begins to exercise, his or her muscles start contracting and demanding more oxygen. Cardiac output must therefore increase, so that more oxygen-rich blood can reach the muscles. The more vigorously the individual exercises, the higher his or her cardiac output becomes. An average person's cardiac output can reach a level of roughly 23 to 26 quarts of blood per minute, while the cardiovascular system of a trained athlete who is exercising strenuously can circulate more than 30 quarts of blood each minute.

Changes in Heart Rate

The *heart rate*—the number of times the heart beats, or contracts, each minute—also changes during exercise. The average person has a resting heart rate of about 72 to 78 beats per minute.

Heart rate, like cardiac output, increases during exercise. The amount of this increase depends on several factors, including the intensity of the exercise, its duration, the temperature and humidity of the air, and the degree of physical conditioning of the person who is exercising. Consider the intensity and duration of the exercise. A person who does 20 sit-ups in the space of 1 to 2 minutes will experience a small increase in heart rate, but someone who runs a mile in 6 minutes will experience a much greater increase. In terms of the degree of physical conditioning, the heart rate of a well-conditioned person will rise more slowly than that of someone who is out of shape. This is because a well-conditioned heart pumps more blood during each contraction and so needs fewer additional contractions to circulate the required extra blood.

During mild exercise or other activity, heart rates of 90 to 120 beats per minute are common. Moderate exercise produces rates of 110 to 150 beats per minute and very intense exercise can result in rates as high as 220. One well-known test of cardiovascular fitness measures

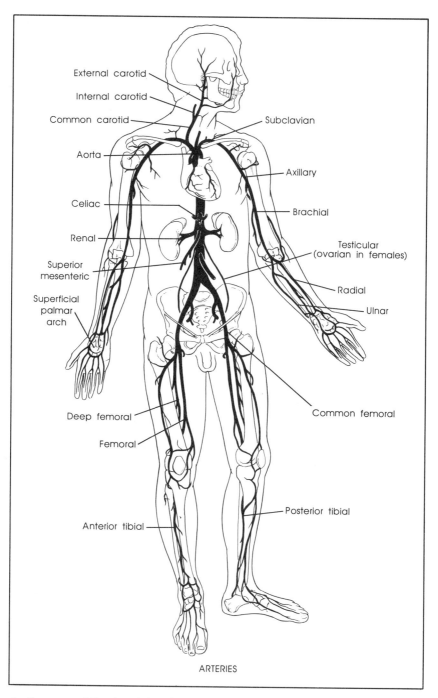

External carotid

Internal carotid

Common carotid

Subclavian

Aorta

Axillary

Celiac

Brachial

Renal

Testicular
(ovarian in females)

Superior
mesenteric

Radial

Superficial
palmar
arch

Ulnar

Deep femoral

Common femoral

Femoral

Posterior tibial

Anterior tibial

ARTERIES

A diagram of the body's arterial system; the arteries transport oxygen-rich blood to muscles and other tissues. An individual's oxygen needs increase dramatically during exercise.

how long it takes for the heart to return to normal after exercise has ceased. The faster the heart returns to its *resting rate,* the healthier it probably is.

When beginning an exercise program, it is important to remember that the heart is a muscle. Like other muscles, it can do only so much work in a given span of time, so care should be taken not to put too much strain upon it, especially if the person exercising is out of shape. On the other hand, the heart needs regular exercise to stay healthy and becomes stronger with increased use. Doing sensible exercises and gradually increasing their intensity and duration over the course of time is the best way to maintain safe and healthy heart function.

THE FLOW OF BLOOD

There are three types of vessels that carry blood through the body: the *arteries,* the *veins,* and the *capillaries.* The arteries transport blood with a high oxygen content to the muscles and other body tissues. There, the blood enters the capillaries, which are only about .00039 inches in diameter and about half an inch long but number in the millions throughout the body. Oxygen from the blood passes through the thin walls of the capillaries and into the cells that make up the tissues. In addition, carbon dioxide and other wastes are discharged by the cells into the capillaries, which empty into the veins. The veins then carry the blood toward the lungs, and the carbon dioxide is removed as the individual exhales.

The heart pumps vigorously to keep blood flowing through all of these vessels. The moving blood pushes on the walls of the vessels, creating pressure, especially in the arteries, which receive the blood directly from the heart. This *blood pressure* is customarily measured in millimeters. That is, millimeters of mercury, since the device used to measure blood pressure, the *sphygmomanometer,* includes a thermometerlike tube filled with mercury. A doctor finds a patient's blood pressure level by reading the level of mercury in the tube. The pressure is recorded twice: once when the heart contracts and arterial pressure is highest (*systolic* pressure), and again between contractions, when

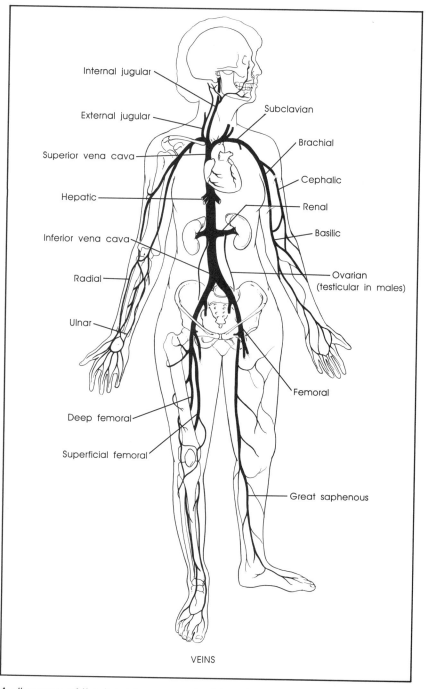

Internal jugular

External jugular

Superior vena cava

Hepatic

Inferior vena cava

Radial

Ulnar

Deep femoral

Superficial femoral

Subclavian

Brachial

Cephalic

Renal

Basilic

Ovarian
(testicular in males)

Femoral

Great saphenous

VEINS

A diagram of the body's venous (vein) system; these blood vessels carry oxygen-poor blood to the lungs, where carbon dioxide is removed from the circulatory system when an individual exhales, and oxygen is replaced when he or she inhales.

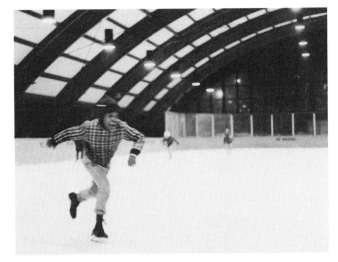

The heart rate rises during exercise in order to meet the body's increased demand for oxygen-rich blood.

arterial pressure is lowest (*diastolic* pressure). Normal blood pressure for a resting adult is about 120 millimeters of mercury over 80 millimeters of mercury, or 120/80.

Because the heart pumps faster during exercise, and thus increases cardiac output, it is not surprising that blood pressure also increases during heightened activity. Such changes are temporary, and blood pressure rapidly returns to normal levels when a person stops exercis-

The trachea and lungs are components of the respiratory system, which is responsible for supplying the blood with oxygen and removing carbon dioxide from the body.

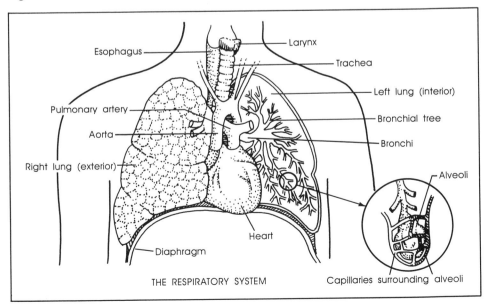

Esophagus

Larynx

Trachea

Left lung (interior)

Pulmonary artery

Bronchial tree

Aorta

Bronchi

Right lung (exterior)

Alveoli

Heart

Diaphragm

THE RESPIRATORY SYSTEM

Capillaries surrounding alveoli

PERFORMING ONE'S OWN CARDIOVASCULAR TEST

Measuring cardiovascular fitness helps an individual determine the amount of work needed to get in shape. There are a number of ways to test endurance, each designed to monitor the cardiovascular system's reaction to some activity. These range from a 12-minute combination of running and walking to the Harvard step test, a 5-minute exercise in which the participant steps up and down again and again, using a small platform. For individuals over age 35, a physician may perform a very sophisticated cardiovascular examination, hooking the patient up to pulse rate and blood pressure monitors and recording these while the person jogs on a treadmill or pedals a stationary bicycle. For a quick and easy way to make a rough endurance estimate, however, the following information may help:

Find the pulse rate, which reflects the rate at which the heart pumps blood through the arteries. Simply place the fingertips of the right hand against the inner part of the left wrist and feel for the rhythmic beat of the blood flowing through the *radial artery*. Count the beats while looking at a clock or watch and find the number of beats that occur within a 10-second period. Multiply by six, and the resulting number is the pulse rate for one minute. The average rate for men is about 72 to 76 beats per minute and for women about 74 to 78. Trained athletes may find that their pulse rate is slower than average, perhaps 60 or below. This is normal and generally nothing to worry about.

Next, run in place for two minutes, making sure to lift the feet at least eight inches from the floor. At the end of the exercise, take the pulse rate again. It will probably be in the 120 to 160 range.

Rest six minutes and then take the pulse rate one more time. If the cardiovascular system is in good condition, the pulse rate

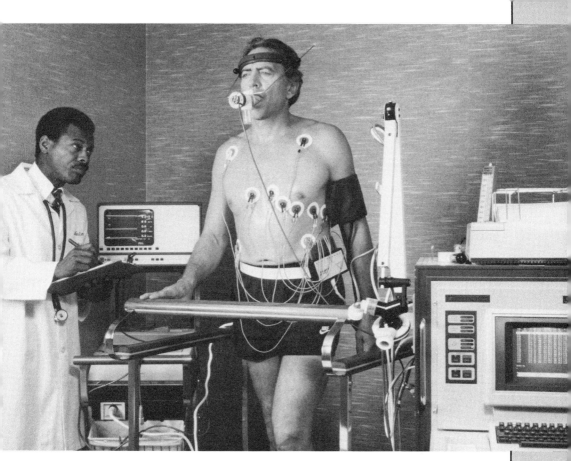

Doctors may use a sophisticated treadmill device to monitor a patient's pulse rate and blood pressure. However, novice exercise enthusiasts can use a much simpler technique to measure cardiovascular fitness.

should have returned to normal (that is, if the rate before running in place was 76, it should be about 76 again). However, if the rate is noticeably higher at this point, cardiovascular fitness may need improvement.

Once an individual has begun a regular exercise program, this test can be taken periodically to measure his or her progress. An important word of warning, how-ever: Older, sedentary individuals or people with certain medical problems, including a history of high blood pressure, coronary artery disease, or problems with the bones, muscles, tendons, or ligaments of the lower limbs should not try this test without a physician's approval.

ing. Too sharp an increase in blood pressure can be dangerous for the body, potentially resulting in broken arteries or, particularly in older people, stroke. This is one reason that exercise should never be too strenuous. Also, people whose resting blood pressure readings are already abnormally high should be especially cautious when exercising. They should perform only moderately difficult exercises and keep workout periods relatively short. To be safe, people with high blood pressure should consult a doctor before starting an exercise program.

EXERCISE AND RESPIRATION

The respiratory system, the major components of which are the *trachea* and lungs, supplies the blood with oxygen and also removes carbon

Breathing is controlled by a muscular wall known as the diaphragm, which expands to pull air into the lungs and contracts to push carbon dioxide out.

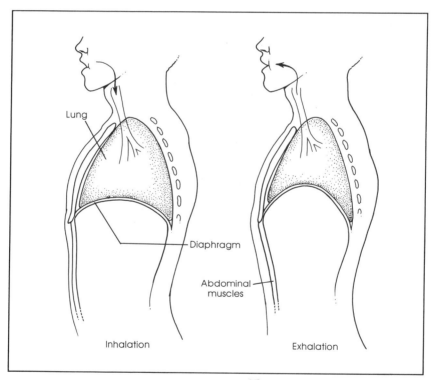

Lung

Diaphragm

Abdominal
muscles

Inhalation

Exhalation

dioxide from the body. The body cannot store oxygen as it stores the nutrients from food. Therefore, although a person can go for perhaps a week or more without food, he or she can normally survive for only about a minute or two without oxygen. This is why the respiratory system is constantly working, even during sleep.

The trachea is a hollow tube through which the air a person breathes passes in order to reach the lungs. Once inside the lungs, the air moves through a system of smaller tubes called *bronchi,* which, in turn, lead to thousands of tiny air sacs known as *alveoli.* The thin walls of the alveoli allow oxygen from the air to pass into the bloodstream. At the same time, the sacs receive carbon dioxide from the blood and this unwanted gas leaves the body when a person exhales. The diaphragm, as mentioned earlier, is an important part of this process, expanding to pull air into the lungs and contracting to push carbon dioxide out.

During exercise, the muscles require a great deal more oxygen than they do when the body is at rest. The more strenuous the exercise, the more oxygen the body needs. Because respiration is the process that brings oxygen into the body, the breathing process is a vital factor in exercise.

When exercise begins, there is an immediate increase in the *minute volume of ventilation,* the amount of air breathed in and out per minute. The higher the minute volume, the more oxygen introduced into the bloodstream and, in turn, carried to the muscles. In very vigorous exercise, the minute volume can expand to as much as 10 times its resting level. Eventually, when the activity becomes too strenuous, the person exercising experiences *dyspnea,* the feeling of being out of breath, and is unable to continue.

Surprisingly, being out of breath has little to do with the breathing process itself. Even at the height of intense exercise, a person is breathing hard enough to pull an adequate supply of oxygen into his or her lungs. Once the oxygen reaches the bloodstream, however, it must pass through the heart, the arteries, and finally the capillaries before it can reach the muscles. This conveyerlike system can only work so fast. In other words, there is a limit to how quickly the body can process the incoming oxygen and get it to the tissues. So, during strenuous exercise, even though the lungs are inhaling large amounts of air, not all of the oxygen in that air is getting to the muscle tissues, and dyspnea sets in.

Second Wind

Some people report that, at times, when they are exercising strenuously and their breathing has become very labored, they suddenly experience a feeling of relief and a renewed ability to continue the activity. This experience is often referred to as getting a *second wind*. During this

Oxygen diffuses from the alveoli (groups of air sacs in the lungs) into the bloodstream. Here it attaches to hemoglobin, protein molecules found in red blood cells. (The oxygen-hemoglobin combination is oxyhemoglobin.) At the same time, hemoglobin releases carbon dioxide to be exhaled through the lungs.

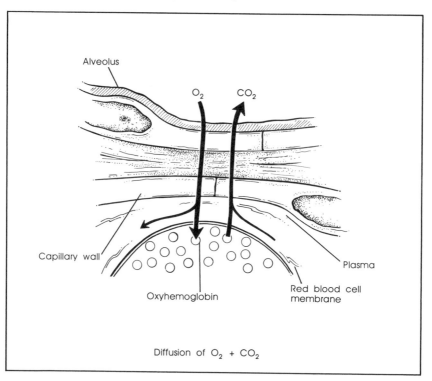

Alveolus

O_2 CO_2

Capillary wall

Plasma

Oxyhemoglobin

Red blood cell membrane

Diffusion of O_2 + CO_2

period, the individual has less trouble breathing, feels less muscle pain, and experiences a more regular heart rhythm. A widely accepted theory suggests that a second wind occurs when, during the early phase of a workout, the muscles reach their most efficient temperature and, at the same time, the body starts redirecting blood from other areas to the skeletal muscles, which in turn helps the muscles work more effectively.

HEART-LUNG ENDURANCE AND GOOD HEALTH

When an individual exercises vigorously on a regular basis, his or her cardiovascular and respiratory systems must continually operate at a more strenuous level than usual. As a result, over time, the heart becomes stronger, is able to pump more blood, and, therefore, can supply more oxygen to the tissues. In addition, regular exercise keeps the blood vessels and lungs in good working order, enhancing their ability to work with the heart and muscles. All of these body components expand their capacity to endure increasing amounts of sustained physical activity. Thus, regular exercise improves both cardiovascular and respiratory endurance and helps keep a person physically fit.

Studies have shown repeatedly that people who are physically fit are healthier and better able to maintain their good health as they grow older. In addition, exercise can keep the body working efficiently well into old age. Many people used to assume that it was chronological age that determined the capacity for exercise. In other words, the older a person got, the less physical exercise he or she could perform. Scientists now know that this is not the case. They have demonstrated that most people can practice sensible, quite vigorous exercise programs even into their seventies and eighties.

In fact, there is considerable evidence that lack of exercise is one of the reasons that the cardiovascular system suffers degenerative diseases, which can strike people in their thirties and forties as well as in later years. The most common and perhaps most devastating example is a weakening of the heart and subsequent heart attack. The less exercise the heart gets, the less strain it can endure. A person with low cardiovascular endurance runs a high risk of heart attack. If that individual also smokes, eats the wrong foods, or has a history of heart disease in his or her family, the risk may increase. By contrast, a person who exercises regularly, does not smoke, and avoids unhealthy foods is probably less likely to suffer a heart attack, regardless of age.

CHAPTER 4

EXERCISE TYPES
AND SKILLS

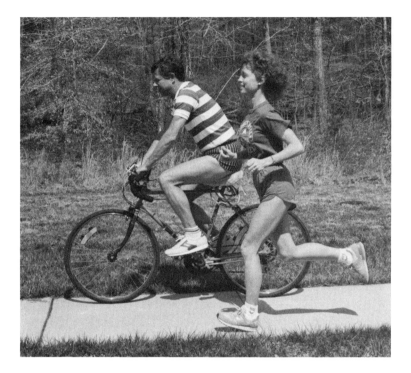

Exercises fall into several different categories. Although they all have the general goal of achieving muscular or cardiovascular fitness, each type approaches the task in a different manner, emphasizing a specific kind of movement or working the muscles in a certain way. One category of exercise can be more effective than another in preparing for a specific sport or other physical activity. Regular aerobic workouts are designed to improve cardiovascular endurance and breathing control. Such exercises are an excellent way to build up to a program of jogging, which is itself an aerobic activity. Personal preference is an important factor in fitness, for sustaining a person's interest in exercise over the course of months or years is sometimes difficult. Some people stick with one type of exercise simply because they prefer it over other types, and others periodically switch from one exercise to another, lessening the chance that they will eventually get bored and quit.

ISOMETRICS

Isometric exercises are those in which the muscles encounter enough resistance to prevent much, if any, movement. An example would be a person pushing against a wall. The muscles of the upper body contract, but the wall offers too much resistance and no movement occurs.

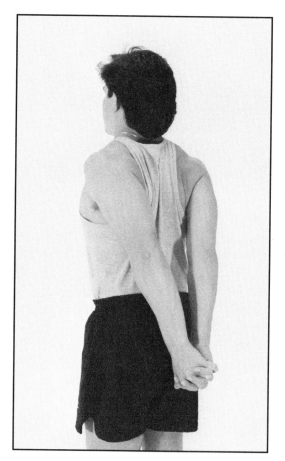

Isometric exercises, such as this one designed to strengthen the back muscles, are performed by forcing muscles to work against each other or to contract against an immovable object.

Medical researchers have long noticed that active children push and pull on immovable objects quite often when playing. This is one of the ways the growing body develops proper muscle tone.

Isometric training for athletes became very popular in the 1950s and 1960s. One common exercise involved standing in a doorway and pressing outward on the doorframe with both hands. An individual exerted maximum force, tightly contracting the muscles of the arms, shoulders, and chest for perhaps 6 to 10 seconds. This procedure was repeated several times before going on to another isometric exercise that used different muscles, such as sitting sideways in the doorframe and pushing against one side with the feet.

Isometric exercises have benefits as well as drawbacks. There is no doubt that isometrics build strength and are beneficial to health. In addition, they are not time-consuming and require no special equipment. However, isometrics do not significantly develop either muscular or cardiovascular endurance. This means that these exercises are mainly good for athletes who want to develop strength in specific muscle groups for use in activities that feature short bursts of strenuous physical exertion. Discus throwers, shot-putters, golfers, bowlers, and baseball pitchers all may benefit from some form of isometric exercise. Isometrics are not particularly helpful in training for sports and activities that require exertion over longer periods of time, such as tennis, basketball, soccer, and jogging.

ISOTONICS

Isotonic exercises are those in which the muscles encounter and overcome resistance, allowing body parts to move. For example, a person lifting a barbell works many of the same muscles as someone pushing against a doorframe. The difference is that the barbell moves, so the person's joints and muscles experience the force of resistance over a much wider range of positions.

The most familiar isotonic exercises are those involved in weight lifting, either with free weights or with weight machines. Both approaches offer a wide range of activities, and the weights can be varied to suit the strength and level of conditioning of the individual.

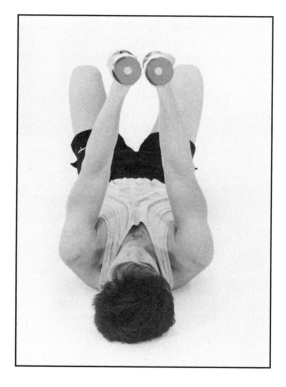

Like isometrics, isotonic exercises are also designed to increase strength, but in this case muscle contractions are used to produce movement.

As previously mentioned, lifting heavier weights for a relatively low number of repetitions, or "reps," tends to develop muscular strength, whereas using lighter weights for a higher number of repetitions tends to improve muscular shape and definition.

CALISTHENICS

Calisthenics are isotonic-type exercises performed without equipment and repeated many times in succession. These include toe touches, push-ups, sit-ups, and jumping jacks. Calisthenics are usually associated with formal training routines such as those used in the military or on high school and college athletic teams. Normally, a person does such exercises in unison with teammates and following the verbal commands of a coach or exercise leader.

Like other forms of exercise, calisthenics have advantages as well as drawbacks. Medical studies have found that regular calisthenics,

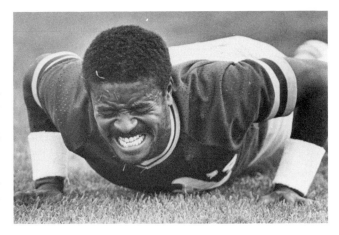

Calisthenics, such as push-ups, are isotonic-type exercises performed without equipment and repeated many times in succession. Regular calisthenics can maintain existing muscle strength but are not very effective at increasing it.

especially strenuous ones such as push-ups, are valuable in maintaining existing muscular strength. By themselves, however, calisthenics are not particularly effective in building strength.

One definite advantage of calisthenics is that they involve a lot of stretching of the muscles and *ligaments,* the tough bands of tissue that connect one bone to another. Therefore, the exercises improve flexibility. One unquestioned disadvantage of calisthenics is that they are monotonous, which means they require a great deal of discipline and dedication. Unfortunately, many individuals who try to get into shape using calisthenics alone quickly become bored and stop exercising entirely. Most fitness authorities advocate using calisthenics in conjunction with other forms of exercise.

AEROBICS

The term *aerobics,* which means "in the presence of oxygen," is relatively new in relation to exercise and athletics, having gained widespread popularity in the 1970s. However, aerobic-type exercises have been practiced for hundreds or even thousands of years. Running, swimming, and cycling are all forms of aerobic exercise if they are performed continuously for a specific period of time.

These activities are designed to develop and improve cardiovascular endurance. Most experts define an aerobic exercise as one that requires at least a moderate amount of exertion and can be continued for a span of five minutes or more without causing fatigue. (Very intense exercises that produce fatigue early on, such as a 100-yard run, are called *anaerobic* activities. Anaerobic means "without oxygen.")

The strenuousness of an aerobic activity can be measured by how much an individual perspires and how high his or her pulse rate rises during the workout. It is generally desirable to raise the pulse rate to between 120 and 150 beats per minute (depending on a person's age) and maintain that level throughout the workout. Often, four to five minutes into the exercise, an individual will begin to perspire. Breaking a sweat is not only an expected part of aerobics but also a good gauge of the effectiveness of the workout. If a person does not sweat, chances are the exercise is not strenuous enough to be truly effective.

Aerobics improve cardiovascular endurance by continually forcing that system to work much harder than it usually does, thereby increasing its efficiency. This measurable improvement is sometimes referred to as the *training effect.* Generally speaking, the longer a person continues an aerobic exercise beyond the five-minute mark, the more extensive the training effect. Performing aerobic workouts lasting 15 to 20 minutes or more is an especially effective method of exercising the cardiovascular system.

In addition to the previous examples, other aerobic activities include running in place, power walking, handball, racquetball, basketball, squash, ice skating, soccer, and cross-country skiing.

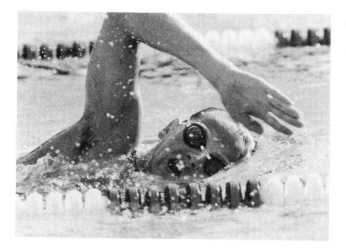

Aerobic exercises, such as swimming, develop and improve cardiovascular endurance.

SKILLS AND LIMITATIONS

Each type of exercise, sport, or other physical activity requires specific skills. For example, gymnastics need balance and flexibility, and hitting a baseball involves *eye-muscle coordination* and timing. Every person's physical makeup is unique, and some people can master certain skills better than others can. A few individuals are blessed with a wide range of skills, and they are the ones who become renowned athletes. Yet even a person with more modest natural physical abilities can, to some degree, develop and improve the skills he or she possesses through regular exercise.

Weight

There are many factors that limit the effectiveness of one's skills. One of the most obvious is body weight. People who are overweight tend to have more difficulty performing most exercises than people of *ideal weight.* An individual's ideal weight is that which medical researchers have determined is healthiest for his or her particular height, build (light, medium, or heavy), and gender. A male who is 5 feet, 7 inches tall with a medium build should ideally weigh about 147 to 150 pounds, while a female who is 5 feet, 2 inches tall with a heavy build should weigh roughly 124 to 127 pounds. If these people actually weigh 180 and 160 pounds respectively, the extra fat content of their body forces them to expend much more effort during exercise than would be necessary at their ideal weight. Simply stated, their heart-lung system and muscles must work particularly hard to accommodate the extra pounds, and they tire much more quickly. Also, the excess weight limits their flexibility and balancing skills.

Height

A relatively short person does not need to move his or her body parts as far as a taller, longer-limbed individual does in order to complete a physical action. Therefore, shorter people have an advantage in physical activities that demand small, measured movements, such

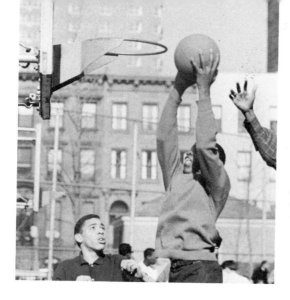

Training can help people of even modest abilities become better at a sport, but height, weight, and muscle mass are important too. Exceptional height, for example, can be a great advantage in basketball.

as climbing, diving, and many gymnastic events. By contrast, taller people have the advantage in exercises that call for larger, more elongated movements. For example, in throwing a baseball or a javelin, more distance and accuracy are possible when the throwing arm moves through a longer curve, or arc. Therefore, a tall person with a long reach often has a great advantage when playing basketball.

An individual's *center of gravity,* another height-related factor, also plays a part in sports skills. The center of gravity is the spot in a person's body where the majority of weight is centered. In shorter individuals, the center of gravity is closer to both the ground and the bases of support (the legs) than it is in taller people. As a result, someone with a low center of gravity can more easily throw a taller person off balance. This is why most champion high school and collegiate wrestlers tend to be short.

Muscle Mass

Physical ability is also affected by the amount of *muscle mass* a person possesses—that is, the actual size of the muscle tissues. Generally speaking, people with larger muscles can lift more weight, exert more pressure, or overcome more resistance than people with smaller muscles. This is why athletes with heavy musculatures are usually the most successful at sports that emphasize strength, such as weight lifting, discus throwing, and football.

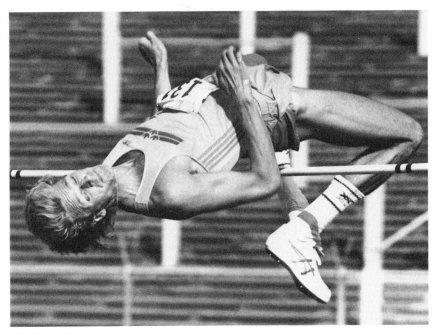

Although heavy muscle mass can be extremely important in such sports as football and weight lifting, a lean build provides a greater advantage for high jumpers fighting against the pull of gravity.

By comparison, heavy muscle mass can be a disadvantage in activities where flexibility or overcoming the pull of gravity are more important. Divers and dancers, who must be able to bend and twist with great dexterity, invariably have lean builds. Tumblers and high jumpers tend also to be lean because heavier builds would weigh them down.

Timing and Coordination

Timing is another factor that affects how well a person can perform a given activity. There are two general aspects of timing. The first is concerned with judgment, knowing exactly when to move an arm or contract a muscle in order to perform the activity most effectively. A baseball batter must be able to sense the precise moment to swing the bat or else he or she will miss the ball, and a tennis player must be able to estimate accurately how fast to run and how far to extend the racket only a second or so after an opponent has hit the ball. These abilities are controlled by the central nervous system. Although it is possible to improve one's timing through diligent practice, some people have a more highly developed nervous system and so have better natural timing.

Reaction time, the amount of time required to respond to a given stimulus, is also an important part of physical ability. Individuals with fast reaction times are sometimes said to have quick reflexes. In some activities, quick reflexes are vital. The sprinter who responds first to the starter's gun has a better chance of winning the race. By contrast, long-distance runners begin at a more leisurely pace and do not need a fast reaction time. Some people are born with quicker reflexes than others and, unfortunately, reaction time cannot be improved. With practice, however, a person can slightly increase the speed with which he or she moves.

One of the most important exercise skills, and one that is related to timing, is eye-muscle coordination. This is the ability of the brain to guide the muscles and other body parts according to a precise pattern based on images received by the eyes. Consider the tennis player mentioned earlier. As the player nears the approaching ball, the visual image of the ball is relayed to the brain. The brain processes the image, then orders the muscles to swing the racket so that it will intercept the ball. All this relaying and processing takes only a fraction of a second. Good eye-muscle coordination is essential to mastering almost every physical activity. Exercises that constantly repeat a certain action will readily improve this skill until it becomes second nature.

Balance and Flexibility

The ability to maintain one's balance is crucial in exercises and sports events of all types, but it is especially so in activities in which the center of gravity and position of the head are constantly shifting and tilting. Jumping, diving, and gymnastic events, as well as dancing, running, skating, wrestling, and boxing all require a highly developed sense of balance.

This sense originates in the inner ear, where tiny physical changes occur when the head and torso tilt. Signals from the inner ear are sent to the brain, which controls the body accordingly. For example, if the body tilts suddenly and unexpectedly, the brain reacts to these changes by signaling the muscles to correct the situation and bring the head or body back to an upright position. When the inner ear is not functioning properly, however, balance is impaired. This is easily demonstrated by an experiment in which a blindfolded athlete stands on a platform. When the platform is tilted, the athlete senses the change and adjusts his or her body position. However, when a hearing-impaired athlete is put in the same situation, he or she is unable to properly sense the increasing tilt and often falls.

During prolonged, rapid head movements, however, the inner ear becomes overstimulated, causing dizziness. An example is the rapid spinning in place performed by both dancers and skaters. These people are able to overcome the feeling of imbalance and nausea by fixing their eyes on a distant object and repeatedly focusing in on that object as they spin. This allows the turning head to rest momentarily during each rotation and thus reduces dizziness.

Flexibility is important in exercises such as calisthenics and dance, and in sports such as gymnastics and swimming, as well as in many everyday activities. An individual's degree of flexibility is determined by the length of and the amount of stretch in the tissues surrounding

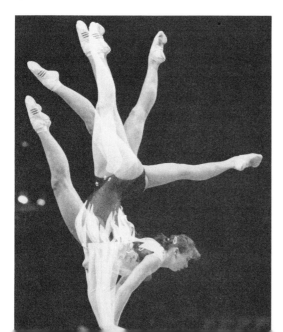

Good balance and flexibility provide a crucial advantage in sports, particularly when an activity requires both the center of gravity and position of the head to constantly tilt and shift.

the joints. The longer and more elastic these tissues are, the more the joints are able to move and the more flexible the body is.

Some of the factors that affect flexibility are bone structure (short, thick bones are less flexible), the amount of stretch in the ligaments, the amount of fat accumulated around the joints (the more fat, the less the joints can move), and the temperature of the air (the joints are more flexible on warmer days).

The best way to develop flexibility is to do regular stretching exercises. The body part being worked should be stretched in one direction only, however, and it is best to go through the motions smoothly, avoiding "bouncing" movements. By extending slightly beyond the point of initial discomfort, the joints and ligaments slowly become more pliable.

A SENSIBLE APPROACH TO EXERCISE

A sensible exercise program does not aim for goals that are unrealistic or physically dangerous. Someone who is 50 pounds overweight will not be able to develop the degree of flexibility that would be possible at his or her ideal weight. If the person forces a body part to stretch too far, muscle strains or torn ligaments can result. Therefore, stretching exercises should not be too rigorous until much or all of the weight is lost.

Often, people exercise too hard because they are trying to emulate someone else. However, they should not despair if they cannot seem to develop the speed, strength, timing, and coordination of a champion. Although such athletes gained a certain amount of their abilities from hard work in the gym or on the field, a major portion of their skills are often a matter of natural talent and body build. These physically gifted individuals represent an extreme minority in any society: No amount of exercise can transform a physically average person into a gifted one. The best course of action for the average person is to select the type of exercise that seems to work best, keep body weight as close to ideal as possible, and try to improve physical skills within reason. Remember that, for most people, the most satisfying long-term goals of fitness are good health and personal enjoyment.

CHAPTER 5

THE IMPORTANCE
OF NUTRITION

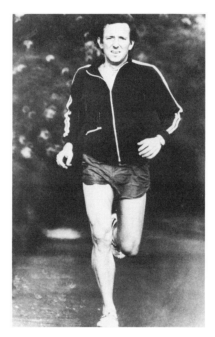

*When jogging guru Jim Fixx suf-
fered a fatal heart attack at
age 52, a poor diet and a previous smoking habit may have
contributed.*

Good nutrition is essential to fitness because of the role nutrients play in maintaining muscles and other body tissues. In addition, consuming certain foods, such as those high in fat, can be harmful to the body. The best exercise program in the world cannot ensure good health for a person with a consistently poor diet. A well-known example is the late Jim Fixx, who wrote a best-selling book about the health advantages of jogging. Fixx had exercised faithfully for years but suffered a fatal heart attack at age 52 while jogging in 1984. Some people said this proved that running, and perhaps exercise in general, is not as good for the heart as exercise advocates claim.

However, experts showed that running itself was not the cause of Fixx's death. There had been a history of heart disease in his family, and Fixx himself was a former smoker, which means that his risk of heart attack may have been higher than that of an average person. Moreover, Fixx reportedly continued to eat foods rich in *cholesterol,* a white, waxy substance found in all animal tissue. Cholesterol tends to accumulate in the arteries, restricting the flow of blood to and from the heart and often, in turn, leading to heart attack. This indicates that a poor diet can greatly reduce the benefits of even the most serious, disciplined exercise program.

HOW THE BODY USES FOOD

With the help of various digestive enzymes and other chemicals, the digestive system breaks food into its basic components, nutrients that travel, via the bloodstream, to the cells, where more chemical reactions take place. In this way, nutrients are used to produce energy to fuel muscle movements. When an individual takes in more nutrients than his or her body needs, the extra materials can be stored as fat and used later. This is why reducing one's food intake results in weight loss. When a person eats less, the body literally transforms some of its own mass into energy for the muscles to use.

Nutritional energy is measured in *calories,* tiny units based on the amount of heat or energy a food is capable of producing in the body. (When the muscles burn energy, heat is produced and the muscles get warmer.) If a relatively small amount of a certain food contains many calories, that food is said to be *highly caloric* or fattening. For example, mayonnaise, which has a high fat content, contains about 100 calories per tablespoon. By contrast, a large, fresh apple contains about 100 calories and is more filling and has much less fat than mayonnaise. Lettuce is also relatively nonfattening. An entire head of iceberg lettuce, enough for several salads, contains only about 40 calories.

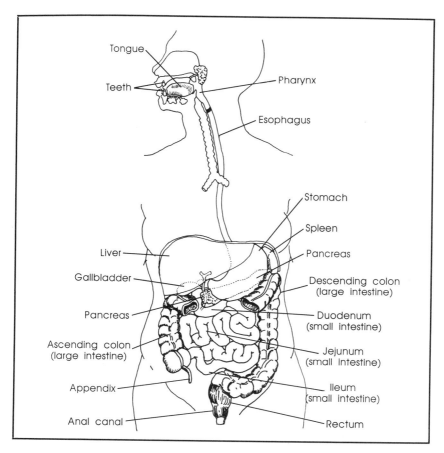

With the help of enzymes and other chemicals, the digestive system breaks food into its basic components, allowing nutrients to travel through the bloodstream to feed cells throughout the body.

EXERCISE AND CALORIES

There is a vital relationship between calorie intake and exercise that helps to determine whether a person will be underweight, overweight, or of ideal weight. The more a person exercises, the more the muscles work and the more nutrients, and calories, are burned. Therefore, exercise is useful in controlling body weight.

Consider an average male, about five feet, six inches tall. If he is fairly inactive, getting little or no exercise, he needs about 1,700 to 2,000 calories per day to keep his body functioning normally. If he is actually consuming that many calories each day, his weight will remain the same. Now suppose that he suddenly increases his food intake to 3,000 calories per day but remains as inactive as ever. His cells now receive many more nutrients than they need, and they store the added calories as fat, causing the man to gain weight. Since 1 pound of weight gain or loss is equivalent to about 3,500 calories, and he is consuming about 1,200 extra calories each day, he can expect to gain about a pound every 3 days.

An increase in the man's level of activity changes the situation somewhat. Suppose that his food intake continues to be 3,000 calories daily but he begins an exercise program that burns 500 calories per day. The man now converts 500 of his 1,200 extra daily calories into heat energy during exercise, which means he stores only 700 calories a day as fat. In that way, although he will continue to add pounds, he will do so at a slower rate.

In order to avoid gaining any weight the man has 2 choices: He can increase the duration of his exercise workouts so that he burns off the entire 1,200 extra calories per day, or he can reduce his daily food

This chart lists the number of calories burned per hour while participating in a variety of sports. Those activities marked with an asterisk are followed by the number of calories burned per mile. However, all the values listed can vary slightly from one person to the next, depending on an individual's gender, weight, and metabolic rate.

How Many Calories Do You Burn During Different Activities?

Aerobic dance	600		Handball	600
Basal metabolism	70		Horseback riding	200-600
Baseball	300		Ice hockey	930
Basketball	500		Rowing *	65-85
Bicycling *	50		Running *	100
Calisthenics	300		Skating	300-700
Canoeing *	75-100		Soccer	550
Cross-country skiing *	100		Squash	600
Downhill skiing	600		Swimming *	400
Field hockey	550		Tennis	500
Football	600-900		Volleyball	210
Golf	300		Walking *	100
Gymnastics	200-500		Weight lifting	500

Source: American Running and Fitness Association (Bethesda, MD)

intake by 1,200 calories. An exercise program that burns 500 calories per day is already on the rigorous side for an average person, so more than doubling the physical exertion in the workouts would probably be too strenuous and do more harm than good. Therefore, in this case, the man should opt for eating less. If he does so, he will still be consuming 500 more calories per day than when he was inactive. The difference is that he will now be burning off those added calories through exercise. The man benefits in two ways. First, he can enjoy the luxury of eating more and still maintain a fixed weight. And second, his exercise program will develop his cardiovascular system.

Now consider an average woman, about five feet, four inches tall, who is very active. She consumes about 2,300 calories per day, the amount she needs to maintain her body weight of 115 pounds. To improve her health, she decides to begin jogging three times a week, but her weight begins to drop. The woman calculates that she is burning about 2,000 calories a week through jogging. As long as her food intake and level of activity remain the same, she will lose more than half a pound a week. Because she prefers not to lose the weight, she has a choice to stop exercising or to start eating more. Since jogging is good for her cardiovascular system and general health, her best choice is to stabilize her weight by increasing her food intake by about 2,000 calories per week. That is only about 300 calories per day, the equivalent of a medium bowl of cereal with milk.

It should now be clear that people who are beginning an exercise program should first decide whether they want to gain, lose, or maintain weight. They can then examine and regulate their average daily calorie intake, adjusting it by factoring in their calorie losses from exercise and other physical activity.

Computing Calorie Requirements

Calculating the number of calories needed per day is relatively easy. First, one must find out the approximate number of calories needed to maintain his or her present weight. (A general physician or nutritionist should know.) Next, one must compute the approximate number of calories burned per day during exercise or other strenuous activity. The chart on page 64 lists some sample activities and the number of calories each burns per hour. Suppose one's usual workout consists of moderately difficult rowing on a rowing machine for 15 minutes and running in place vigorously for another 15 minutes. Since the rowing burns 660 calories per hour, it burns 165 calories in a quarter of an hour. The 15 minutes of running burns one-quarter of 720 calories, or 180 calories. The total number of calories burned in the half hour workout is 165 plus 180, or 345.

The next step in computing calorie requirements is deciding how much food to eat, which will depend on whether one wants to maintain, gain, or lose weight. If an individual wants to stay at his or her present weight, it will be necessary to increase food intake by about 350 calories per day as long as workouts continue on a regular basis. If weight loss or gain is the goal, calorie intake should be increased or decreased accordingly.

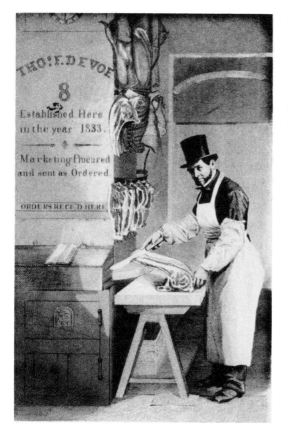

Meat is rich in protein but also tends to be high in fat. Although some fat in the diet is essential to good health, too much can lead to weight gain and an increased risk of heart attack.

COMPONENTS OF FOOD

So far, the discussion has centered on calories. Considered on their own, however, calories are not a reliable gauge of good nutrition. For instance, sugar has very little, if any, nutritional value, yet it does contain calories. Therefore, although a person could conceivably consume nothing but sugar each day and meet his or her calorie requirements, the individual would quickly become weak, dizzy, and malnourished. If this situation continued long enough, the person would die of malnutrition. Thus, maintaining proper nutrition is not just a matter of consuming the right number of calories. Most of those calories should come from nutritious foods.

There are three basic types of food: carbohydrates, proteins, and fats. Foods high in carbohydrates include potatoes, pastas, grains and breads, and most fruits. Some examples of protein-rich foods are lean meat, fish, chicken, eggs, and milk. Vegetables, fruits, and grains also contain protein, although in smaller concentrations. Most foods contain at least some fat, but items such as cream, butter, pork, pastries, and oils are especially high in it. Deciding exactly which foods to eat is a matter of personal choice, but it is essential that the diet include at least some foods from each of the three basic categories. Carbohydrates, proteins, and fats, in varying proportions, are all indispensable to good health.

The desired proportions, or ratios, of these components in the human diet vary from person to person. People who are very active or

Dairy products, such as cheese, are also good sources of protein and contain large amounts of calcium. Like meat, however, they are often high in fat.

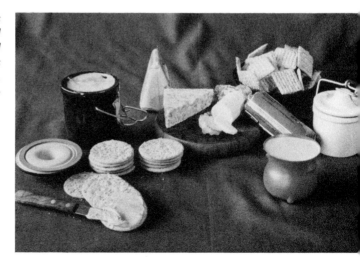

who perform regular, extended aerobic workouts need a higher intake of carbohydrates than less active individuals. This is because active people burn more energy, and the body tissues can readily convert carbohydrates into the fuel they need. This is done via a process called the *Krebs cycle,* a series of reactions that produce energy as well as carbon dioxide (which is exhaled through the lungs) and water (which is eliminated through urine and sweat). Initially, carbohydrates break down into *glucose,* a type of sugar. The body, in turn, breaks glucose down into the chemical *acetyl coenzyme A* (acetyl coA). This then combines with *oxaloacetic acid* to form *citric acid,* and that initiates the Krebs cycle.

For extremely active people, the desired daily food ratio might be 60% to 70% carbohydrate, 10% to 20% protein, and 15% to 20% fat. By contrast, people who are trying to build and maintain muscle mass, such as weight lifters, require a higher intake of protein, which is vital to increasing and maintaining muscle mass. The desired food ratio for these people might be 60% to 70% carbohydrate, 15% to 20% protein, and 15% to 20% fat. These are very general estimates, however.

VITAMINS

Vitamins are complex substances that exist in plant and animal tissue. Small amounts of vitamins are absolutely essential to the normal functioning of the different systems of the body, and severe deficiencies can seriously impair health. A consistent lack of vitamin A can result in rough, peeling skin, night blindness, and loss of color vision. Vitamin C deficiency can leave an individual feeling weak and drowsy and result in *scurvy,* a disease characterized by bleeding under the skin. Obviously, then, getting enough of each vitamin is essential.

Because exercise burns calories and may cause the tissues to utilize vitamins faster than they would normally, people who work out regularly should be especially careful about vitamin intake. Although some individuals must supplement their diet by taking vitamin pills, in most cases this is unnecessary. For a majority of people, minimum daily vitamin requirements can be met by eating enough of certain vitamin-rich foods. For example, there are particularly high amounts of vitamin

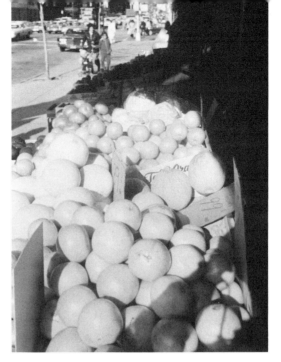

Although under certain conditions vitamin pills can boost health, most people can get all the vitamins they need from their diet. Citrus fruits, for example, are high in vitamin C.

C (also called *ascorbic acid*) in citrus fruits, broccoli, tomatoes, sweet peppers, berries, melons, and potatoes. Generally speaking, maintaining a balanced diet will ensure the proper intake of vitamins and other important nutrients.

MINERALS

Minerals are another basic part of a healthy diet. Although vitamins are considered *organic* substances, which means they contain carbon, minerals are *inorganic,* or non–carbon containing. Important minerals include calcium, phosphorus, magnesium, sodium, potassium, chloride, sulfur, copper, iron, iodine, and zinc. Such substances help the body carry out a variety of functions, including helping to build bones, maintain cell structure, burn fuel, and transport oxygen through the bloodstream.

MAINTAINING A BALANCED DIET

Nutritional experts agree that a balanced diet must provide all the carbohydrates, proteins, fats, vitamins, and minerals necessary for

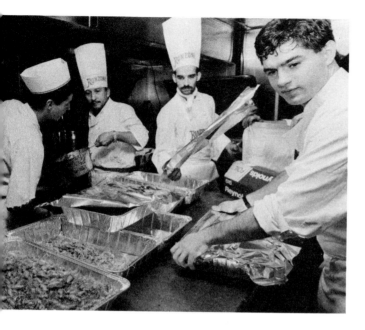

Each year, a pasta party is held prior to the New York City Marathon. Carbohydrates, found in foods such as pastas, potatoes, grains, breads, and fruits, are readily converted by the body into energy, which is a boon to long-distance runners.

good health. However, there is considerable disagreement among experts and the general public alike about which foods should be included in this diet. For instance, vegetarians prefer to exclude meat and sometimes even dairy products (which also come from animals) from their menu. Until recently, many people considered this dietary approach unusual or even potentially unhealthy, believing that meat and dairy products were the only reliable sources of protein and calcium, a mineral important to health. Posters in schools used to emphasize the importance of the *four basic food groups,* which included: 1) nuts and grains, 2) fruits and vegetables, 3) meats, and 4) milk and dairy products.

Studies have shown, however, that all the nutrients necessary for good health, including protein and calcium, are present in plant products—that is, fruits, vegetables, and grains. Plant protein is not as concentrated as the protein found in meat or milk, but eating the right amounts and combinations of vegetables and grains will provide more than enough protein to sustain health. In fact, some experiments suggest that people who eat large amounts of meat and dairy products every day may actually get too much protein, making it more difficult for their digestive system to break down calcium and other important nutrients. This does not mean that people should not eat meat or dairy products, but that they can choose not to and still be healthy. As long as nutritional requirements are met, the kinds of foods consumed are largely a matter of individual preference.

Sometimes, other health factors influence dietary preferences. In recent years, for example, many people besides traditional vegetarians have cut back on or even eliminated their use of meat and dairy products, in an attempt to reduce their intake of cholesterol. Although people need cholesterol—it is essential to the normal functioning of the brain and nervous system—the body manufactures all the cholesterol it needs, and, as mentioned previously, the extra cholesterol absorbed by eating meat and dairy products tends to accumulate on the insides of the blood vessels. In addition to cholesterol, meat and dairy products contain a great deal of fat, which also contributes to the buildup of cholesterol and the onset of heart disease.

As shown here, cholesterol can clog arteries and lead to heart attack. Meats and dairy products tend to be particularly high in cholesterol.

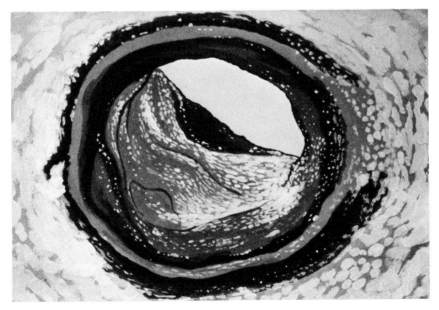

However, there are ways health-conscious individuals can attempt to avoid problems associated with excess cholesterol and fat. These include substantially reducing the amount of meat and dairy products in one's diet, substituting chicken and fish for pork and red meat (which contain more cholesterol per pound), and switching to a diet consisting primarily of fruits, vegetables, and grains. Keeping cholesterol and fat levels low is especially important for people who exercise, because they regularly force their heart and blood vessels to work vigorously. The death of runner Jim Fixx may be a good illustration of just how important the relationship of diet to exercise is to good health.

CHAPTER 6

BEHAVIORS THAT IMPEDE FITNESS

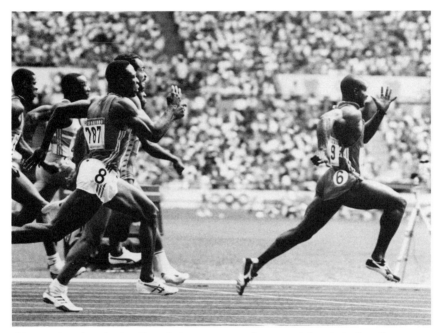

Champion track star Ben Johnson, seen here out front during the 1988 Olympics in Seoul, Korea, was forced to give up his Olympic medal when it was discovered that he had used steroids. Johnson, currently drug free, began a comeback attempt in early 1991.

There are several behaviors, habits, and activities that reduce the effectiveness of exercise and impede fitness. The most destructive are lack of sleep, tobacco use, alcohol consumption, and drug abuse. All of these are damaging to good health and counteract the benefits of regular exercise. Fortunately, each is preventable because in most cases people engage in such behaviors by choice or habit.

LACK OF SLEEP

With rare exceptions, everyone experiences a recurring, approximately 24-hour cycle in which they are awake for so many hours and asleep for the rest. Scientists refer to this pattern as part of the body's *circadian rhythm,* the daily built-in cycles that, among other things, determine what time of day an individual becomes tired and falls asleep. Although researchers are not completely sure why or how the circadian rhythm induces sleep, they have established that one function of sleep is to allow the brain and other body parts to recover from the activity they experience during waking hours. This includes the recovery of the muscle tissues from fatigue brought on by exercise.

A few people are unable to get enough sleep because of a medical condition called *insomnia,* which is basically a difficulty falling or staying asleep and can be caused by such problems as anxiety and depression. Although many individuals can overcome the condition without a doctor's help, others require medical care. Physicians attempt to treat this problem on an individual basis, either with or without drugs.

For the average person, it is normal to have occasional sleeplessness due to excitement, emotional upset, stress, or some other factor. In addition, a rare special event such as a party or the broadcast of a favorite movie on the late, late show may mean sacrificing all or part of a night's sleep. Usually, though, the person immediately resumes a normal schedule.

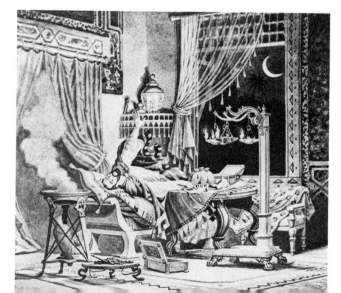

An ancient Roman tossing and turning in bed. The proper amount of sleep is essential to good health. People who continually suffer from insomnia may not only become chronically fatigued but may be less able to resist diseases such as hepatitis and pneumonia.

However, there are some people who, for reasons related either to work or recreation, continually fail to get the amount of sleep their body needs. The consistent loss of sleep over a period of weeks and months results in *chronic fatigue,* a condition in which the body is never allowed to fully recover from the effects of fatigue. The symptoms of this long-lasting problem are difficulty concentrating, sluggishness, poor judgment, short-term memory loss, and reduced ability to deal with stress. In addition, chronic fatigue lowers the body's resistance to diseases such as mononucleosis, hepatitis, and pneumonia, as well as to common allergies.

At the same time, there is no hard-and-fast rule concerning the amount of sleep that should be considered sufficient. Medical experts agree that the old adage about getting eight hours a night does not hold true for everyone. Some individuals function perfectly well on 5 to 6 hours a night, whereas others need 9 to 10 hours a night in order to function normally. People who are exercising regularly will find that

Smoking irritates and clogs air sacs in the lungs, causing short-ness of breath. The problem is particularly bad for people who exercise, because they need a large volume of oxygen to nourish muscle tissue.

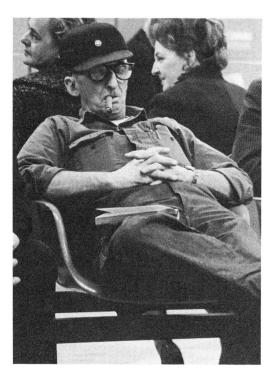

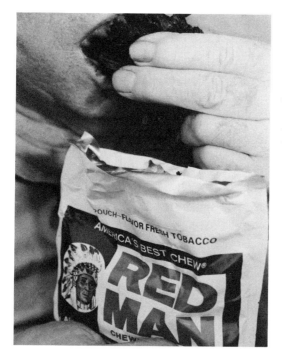

Chewing tobacco is not a safe alternative to cigarettes. About 9,000 Americans die each year from oral cancer, mostly from the use of chewing tobacco.

sleep and exercise reinforce each other. The sleep is necessary for recovery from exercise-induced fatigue and, at the same time, the exercise helps to make sleep patterns more regular and sleep itself deeper and more restful.

TOBACCO USE

Cigarette smoking is the leading cause of preventable illness and death. Each year, more than 300,000 people die of smoking-related illnesses in the United States alone. Cigarette smoke contains *nicotine,* a highly poisonous alkaloid substance; *carbon monoxide,* a toxic gas; and dozens of solid pollutants including *tars* and *hydrocarbons.*

Smoking irritates and clogs the air sacs in the lungs, reducing lung capacity and causing noticeable shortness of breath. This becomes a particular problem for athletes or people who exercise regularly, because they need high amounts of oxygen to replenish muscle tissues. Continued smoking can eventually lead to *emphysema*—a destructive scarring of lung tissue—or to lung cancer.

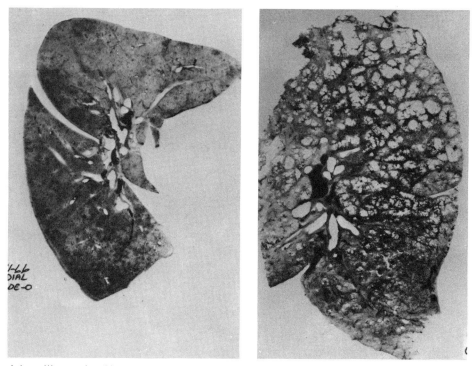

A healthy pair of lungs appears on the left; the effect from years of tobacco smoke can be seen on the right.

Smoking also contributes to the risk of heart disease by speeding up the pulse rate, raising blood pressure, and constricting blood vessels. By weakening the heart-lung system, smoking interferes with cardiovascular training and impairs general fitness.

In addition to being toxic, the nicotine in tobacco is also highly addictive, which makes smoking a difficult habit to break. Therefore, the best way to avoid the health hazards of smoking is never to start smoking in the first place.

Despite its widespread use among athletes, *chewing tobacco* is also an addictive, dangerous substance. About 9,000 Americans die each year from various forms of oral cancer, most of which stem from the use of chewing tobacco. One of the most publicized crises was that of Sean Marsee, a high school senior from Ada, Oklahoma, who began using smokeless tobacco at the age of 13. Despite three operations, he died of oral cancer in 1984.

DRUG USE

Alcohol

The use of alcohol and other drugs can also hinder fitness. Alcohol depresses, or slows, the functions of the brain and nervous system. Studies have shown that, used infrequently and in small amounts, the substance is not harmful to most people. However, like tobacco, alcohol is highly addictive, and it is easy to get into the habit of drinking more often and in greater amounts.

There are many reasons why people who want to develop and maintain health and fitness should not drink too much alcohol. First, the drug has been shown to destroy brain cells that control coordination and reflexes. Alcohol slows reaction time considerably and can also damage nerves in the arms and legs. In addition, heavy alcohol use weakens muscle tissue, a condition particularly noticeable in large muscles, such as those in the legs. The heart, of course, is a muscle and it too can be weakened by repeated, heavy alcohol consumption. Moreover, drinking an unusually large amount of alcohol in one sitting can sometimes cause sudden heart failure. Very heavy and prolonged use of the drug leads to problems such as stomach and intestinal ulcers, internal bleeding, and liver damage.

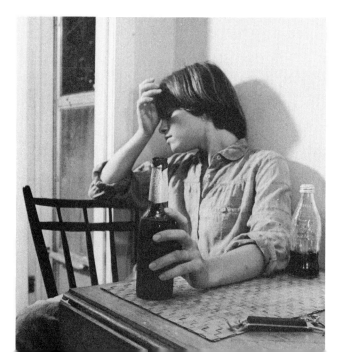

Drug use can contribute to poor health. Alcohol, for example, has been found not only to destroy brain cells but to slow reaction time, damage nerves in the arms and legs, weaken muscle tissue, and cripple the heart and liver.

Marijuana and Cocaine

Other drugs are also physically harmful and thus interfere with health and fitness. Marijuana, a widely used recreational drug, is a *hallucinogen*—a substance that, when taken in large doses, can produce hallucinations. Although smoking marijuana is apparently not physically addicting, it causes most of the same respiratory and cardiovascular damage that cigarette smoking does. Therefore, it is a mistake for those who exercise on a regular basis to think that marijuana use is a safe substitute for tobacco.

Cocaine is a stimulant, a substance that temporarily excites, or speeds up, many body functions. Cocaine, which is usually sniffed, and *crack,* a very pure form of the drug that is often smoked, are both extremely addictive, frequently causing physical and psychological dependence after only a few days of repeated use. Many cocaine users suffer from ulcers and bleeding of the nasal cavity, negative changes in personality, and insomnia. Heavy, prolonged use of the drug damages the spinal cord, causing the user to suffer violent convulsions and making breathing difficult. Death often results.

When someone who exercises regularly becomes a habitual cocaine user, he or she inevitably finds it more and more difficult to maintain a fitness program. The user's judgment is affected by the drug, making accidents and injuries more likely. Breathing is increasingly impaired. The drug can also force the heart to beat irregularly, so that exercise, or any other kind of exertion, can actually become life threatening.

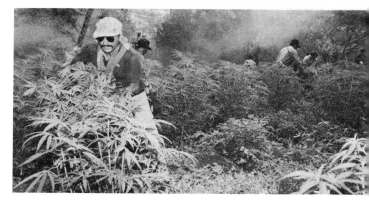

Marijuana, like tobacco, has been found to cause respiratory and cardiovascular damage. Mexican federal police are shown here uprooting marijuana plants near Michoacán, as part of their country's eradication campaign.

Steroids

The use of a very controversial class of drugs, *steroids,* is now wide-spread among athletes in many countries. Steroids are powerful chemicals similar to *testosterone,* the male hormone that maintains secondary sexual characteristics such as a deep voice and facial hair. Steroids have become popular with weight lifters, football players, and other athletes in recent years because the drugs sometimes help to increase muscle mass and, therefore, strength.

However, health experts have shown that steroid use can be dangerous to health. Many people who have used the drugs regularly have developed liver damage and also liver cancers. In addition, steroids adversely affect the cardiovascular system. Repeated steroid use allows cholesterol to build up on the insides of the blood vessels. The consequences are the same as those of improper diet: Blood pressure goes up and the risk of heart attack and stroke increases.

As with tobacco, alcohol, marijuana, cocaine, and other substances that are detrimental to health, the best way to avoid the destructive effects of steroids is never to use them in the first place. Medical researchers agree that avoiding drugs, maintaining a nutritious diet, keeping an approximately ideal weight, and getting sufficient sleep will all make a regular exercise program most effective.

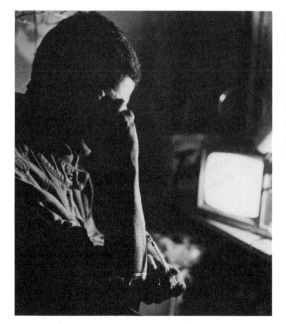

A man injects cocaine at a crack house in the South Bronx, New York. Among its many hazards, the drug can cause irregular heartbeat, turning exercise and other types of exertion into life-threatening activities.

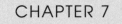

CHAPTER 7

CREATING
A PERSONAL
FITNESS PROGRAM

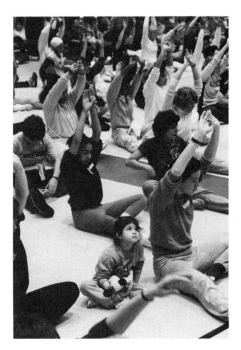

Anyone can develop a successful fitness program by combining safe, sensible exercises with good nutrition and the right amount of sleep. Here are some general guidelines to creating an exercise plan for the person who is out of shape and unaccustomed to regular exercise. Also included is advice on putting together a more advanced program.

INITIAL PREPARATIONS: BEGINNER'S PLAN

The first step in creating a basic exercise regimen is choosing the approach that best suits the individual. This means that the subject must decide what aspects of fitness to emphasize. Some people may want to increase muscular strength, while others might be more interested in improving muscular and cardiovascular endurance. On the other hand, perhaps an individual's goal is to improve the overall flexibility of his or her joints. The healthiest and most beneficial approach is to construct a beginning program that emphasizes all three goals—flexibility, muscular strength, and muscular and cardiovascular endurance. The exercise instructions that follow contain some activities that develop each of these aspects. Later on, in a more advanced program, the subject may concentrate on developing one or two of these.

Although most people can begin exercising any time they wish, it is very important for some individuals to consult a doctor first. People with serious allergies; a history of heart disease, liver, kidney, or respiratory problems; or those who have recently broken bones or suffered other major injuries should seek the advice of a physician before starting any workout program. Most of these individuals will learn that it is safe for them to exercise, but a few will find that they have certain restrictions, and these should be strictly observed.

For those who are completely out of shape, it is important to start slowly and build. One of the biggest mistakes beginners make is to do too much too fast, to work out too long and too strenuously before their body is ready. This usually leads to excessive fatigue, muscle strain, and other injuries, all of which may tempt someone to quit after only a few days or weeks.

The best approach to exercise is to be patient and allow the body to develop at its own pace. Remember that the effects of months and years of physical inactivity cannot be reversed in only a few weeks. The average beginner should plan on a basic program lasting at least two to four months (depending on the individual) before attempting a more advanced workout regimen.

Many beginners find it useful and motivating to record their progress from workout to workout and from week to week on a chart. Such

Pick a Sport!

	Aerobic dance	Basketball	Cross-country skiing	Cycling	Handball/Racquetball	Jogging/Running	Mini-trampoline	Rope skipping	Rowing	Skating	Soccer	Swimming (laps)	Tennis	Walking
For those who are out of shape	●		●	●			●			●	●	●	●	●
For those in great shape	●	●	●	●	●	●		●			●	●		
For those who want to be alone				●		●	●	●	●	●		●		●
For those who like company	●	●			●					●	●	●		
For those who hate to sweat												●		
For those who want to be indoors	●	●	●	●	●	●	●	●	●	●	●	●	●	●
For those who want to be outdoors		●	●	●		●			●	●	●	●	●	●
For those who have problems with their joints			●	●			●		●			●		●
For those who do not have much time	●		●		●	●	●	●						
For those who are easily bored	●	●			●					●			●	
For those who are competitive			●		●	●	●			●	●	●	●	
For those who cannot spend much money			●					●			●			●
For those who want to become more flexible	●		●		●			●		●	●			●
For those who are modest and do not want to wear shorts			●	●		●		●						●

Source: American Running and Fitness Association (Bethesda, MD)

a chart might list the exercises performed, leaving space after each to mark down the number of repetitions performed or the time taken to complete the activity. The chart can be used to create a number of small, individual goals to attain and personal records to beat, as an added incentive to keep exercising.

General Training Tips

Perhaps the single most important aspect of exercise is establishing and maintaining a routine. No matter how enthusiastic the individual, there will be some days when he or she just does not feel like exercising. This is where self-discipline comes in. One way to build discipline and stay on a schedule is to remember what happens after skipping several workouts: The muscles and other body parts begin to revert to their former, unconditioned state and much of the hard work already put in is wasted. Something else to keep in mind is that, although various speeds, distances, and intensities are suggested in some of the exercises described, these are only rough guidelines. It is especially important for a beginner to start with a pace that is manageable and to slow down when he or she becomes out of breath. Older individuals, who generally lead a more sedentary life-style, should take particular care to build gradually to a more strenuous workout.

Scheduling

If the exercise program consists mainly of calisthenics, light aerobics, and other exercises that require minimal exertion, it is normally all right to exercise every day. However, very strenuous workouts should be performed only every other day, to allow the body to rest a day in between. It is also helpful to vary the exercise routine in each workout in order to alternately concentrate on different muscles or body parts. For instance, it is best not to follow one leg exercise with another leg exercise but to instead move on to an activity that works the waist or some other area of the body. That helps prevent an individual from overusing one muscle group. Another benefit is that varying the exercises makes the workout less boring.

Another acceptable approach is to work on a specific muscle group or body area one day and a different group or area the next. For example, an individual could concentrate on the upper body on Mondays, Wednesdays, and Fridays and the lower body on Tuesdays, Thursdays, and Saturdays. It is advisable to take at least one day off from exercise each week.

Breathing

Proper breathing is another important part of exercise. A good general rule is to inhale before beginning an individual rep and to exhale while completing the action. This keeps an adequate supply of oxygen flowing into the lungs and also creates an exercise rhythm that can make repetitions easier to perform.

Pain

Everyone who begins a new exercise program notices soreness in the muscles and joints in the days following the first few workouts. Remember that the muscles of an inactive person react to the sudden increased work load by aching. This pain is completely normal and disappears after a week or two. However, if the strenuousness of the program is suddenly increased or different muscles are worked, the aches and pains will return. Once again, this is to be expected; the discomfort is temporary and nothing to worry about. However, any unusually sharp and localized pain that does not go away in a day or two may indicate a torn muscle or some other injury and should be looked at by a doctor.

The Warm-up

It is extremely important to include a short warm-up session before each full exercise workout. This not only slightly warms the muscles,

A short warm-up session prior to a full workout can help prepare the muscles and increase flexibility. Side bends are an effective way to stretch the waist and lower back.

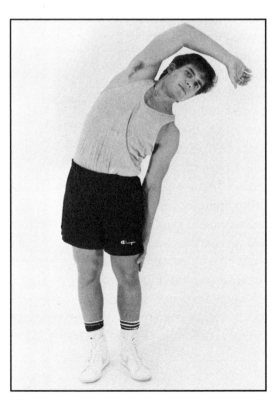

EXERCISE AND INJURY

Despite its many benefits, exercise can cause injury, particularly if an individual does not prepare adequately or use the right equipment. Problems can range from minor aches and pains to serious damage requiring medical treatment. Common examples include the following:

- Numerous types of **back injuries** affect weekend athletes and sports figures alike. For example, trouble may result for an individual if one leg is shorter than the other, a relatively common condition. If the legs differ by more than half an inch and an individual's workout involves a great deal of running, he or she will be continually placing uneven pressure on the spinal column, and possibly causing severe pain. The problem can be avoided by using a shoe insert on the shorter leg. Of course, there are many other examples of back injuries, ranging from the lower back pain caused by leaning over the handles of a racing bike to the slipped disk sometimes incurred in sports such as football and weight lifting. Treatment for back problems, depending upon

their severity, may include rest, some form of therapy, or even surgery.

- **Blisters** are formed by friction against the skin, causing fluid to accumulate beneath the surface. However, they can be avoided by allowing a sensitive area of the body to become toughened through a gradual increase in activity, or by protecting it with the proper covering, such as gloves, extra socks, or bandages.
- **Frostbite** (cold weather damage to the skin) can result when the body is poorly protected against freezing temperatures. Symptoms of frostbite include pale skin and numbness. Treatment includes gradual warming of the frostbitten area. This is best done by immersing it in lukewarm water. (Do not attempt to heat the area by rubbing it; this can actually cause more tissue damage.) In addition, the patient should be quickly taken to an emergency room for further treatment.
- **Heatstroke** can occur while exercising in hot, humid weather and results when the body produces a great deal

more heat than it can release. Symptoms include blurred vision, dizziness, nausea, and fainting spells. Heatstroke can be avoided by consuming six or more glasses of liquid a day, drinking extra water before exercising, and refraining from workouts in extreme heat and humidity. If heatstroke occurs, the victim should be taken out of the sun and allowed to lie down, with the feet higher than the head. Pouring water over the individual or applying a damp cloth is important as well, and the victim should drink water or, if he or she is unable to drink, be given saltwater injections. Medical help is also essential. Without proper care, heatstroke can be fatal.

- **Runner's knee** results from sprained ligaments in the joint and is caused by overuse. A mild sprain in this area can be treated by packing the knee in ice and wrapping an elastic bandage around it. A severe sprain, which may include torn cartilage, a large amount of swelling, and a great deal of pain, should receive quick medical attention.
- **Shinsplints** usually result when tendons attached to muscles in front of the lower leg and the membrane surrounding the shinbone become inflamed. The condition can result from jogging on hard pavement and overuse when individuals first start a running program, or when joggers land on their toes instead of their heels. Exercises to condition the lower leg, landing heel first when running, and wearing a well-cushioned shoe can help prevent the problem. The injury can often be treated by wrapping and resting the legs and by applying ice.
- Severely twisting a joint can cause a **sprain,** resulting in torn ligaments and ruptured blood vessels. The injury most often strikes the knees and ankles and may occur when an individual does not warm up properly before exercising, overworks a tired muscle, or suffers an accident that twists the joint. Sprains can range from minor injuries that cause only a small amount of pain and swelling to a complete tear of a muscle or tendon.

Although the list of sports-related injuries is a long one, it should not intimidate anyone planning to get into shape. It should simply serve to indicate that caution and common sense are an important part of any workout.

making them receptive to more strenuous exertion and less susceptible to injury, but also stretches the joints and ligaments, increasing flexibility and reducing the chance of sprains.

The warm-up should briefly work each major muscle group or body area. For example, leg stretches, performed by placing the sole of the foot against a wall or other vertical surface and pushing the leg forward, loosens and prepares the rear section of the lower leg. Push-ups are good exercises for warming up the upper body. Depending on the individual's level of conditioning, 3 to 10 push-ups are generally sufficient to prepare for a beginner's workout.

Twisting movements, on the other hand, can help prepare the waist and lower back. One should stand with the legs at shoulder width and twist at the waist from side to side, trying each time to turn far enough to see directly behind. However, twisting farther and farther with each rotation could tear a muscle, so it is important not to overdo. *Side bends,* performed by standing and leaning over sideways as far as is comfortable, are also effective for stretching the waist and lower back.

In the case of someone suffering from lower back trouble, a good alternative waist exercise is the *crunch.* This is done by lying faceup on the floor, holding the hands behind the head or the arms crossed over the chest, bending the knees, and placing the feet on the floor or on the edge of a bed, chair, or workout bench. The next step is to lift both the buttocks and the head off the floor so that the body is held up by only the legs and upper back, and exhaling while holding the position for several seconds. Each time this action is repeated, the abdominal muscles will tighten, while the lower back remains relatively relaxed.

However, some stretching exercises may not be completely safe. For example, deep squats can overstretch ligaments in the knee, and traditional toe touches (bending over with both legs straight) can strain the lower back.

A STARTER PROGRAM

The following are some good general exercises for a beginning fitness program. The total number of reps of a specific exercise performed

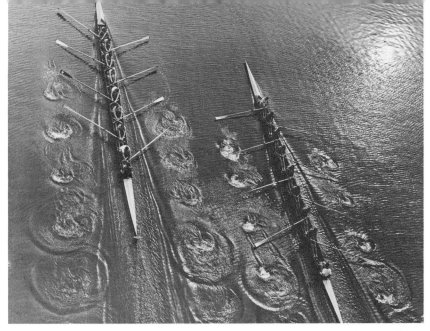

Rowing exercises most upper body muscles and benefits the cardio-vascular system as well.

without interruption is called a *set*. The number of sets and reps in a workout will vary from person to person, depending on the subject's level of conditioning. Those in better shape will be able to do a greater number of sets, with more reps in each set. During the first few weeks of the program, a typical workout might consist of only 1 or 2 sets of each exercise with 5 to 10 reps in each set. However, after two months, the workout could well include three or four sets of each activity with dozens or even hundreds of reps in some sets. The individual must decide on the number of sets and reps that are the safest and most effective and must also know when a workout is too intense. As previously stated, some aches and pains are to be expected, particularly when the workout is increased; however, certain signals can mean that an individual is exercising too strenuously. These include sharp or persistent pain, nausea, dizziness, and extreme shortness of breath. Remember that each workout should be preceded by a warm-up session.

Upper Body Exercises

Push-ups   In addition to doing standard push-ups, it is possible to work different muscles of the upper body in different ways by changing the distance between the hands. Holding the hands closer together emphasizes the rear arm and upper back muscles, but holding the hands farther apart works more on the sides of the chest and the biceps. Inclined push-ups are also effective. These are done by placing the hands on a bed, bench, or chair so that the body is at an angle to the floor.

Isometric pushes and pulls   Simple isometric pushes can be performed by placing the hands together, palm to palm, and forcefully pushing for several seconds. A variation is to stand in a doorway and push against the sides of the doorframe. Placing the hands at varying heights will put emphasis on different muscles. Isometric pulls are executed by interlocking the fingers of the hands and vigorously pulling outward for several seconds. Standing between two poles, grasping the poles, and pulling inward is an effective variation.

Rowing   Rowing, either performed in a boat or using a rowing machine, works most of the muscles of the upper body. During the first few weeks of exercise, the individual should row slowly and methodically, with the aim of building strength and muscular endurance. Later, the person can either greatly increase the number of reps or do as many reps as possible in a given time period, perhaps four minutes. Note that rowing is also an excellent cardiovascular exercise.

Waist and Lower Back Exercises

Sit-ups   Sit-ups can be performed in several ways. Lying on the floor with the legs straight and the feet tucked under a piece of furniture (for

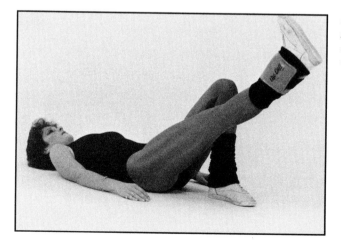

Leg lifts are among a set of exercises aimed at strengthening the waist or lower back.

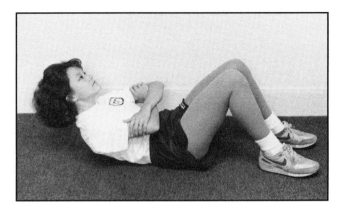

Sit-ups designed to avoid back strain are performed by slowly curling the head and shoulders to a 30-degree angle, holding for 5 seconds, and lowering slowly to the floor.

leverage) is the most common method. Bent-knee sit-ups are more difficult but can be attempted after the first two weeks of exercise. Inclined sit-ups, done lying on a tilted board with the head pointed downward, are quite effective for working the abdominal muscles but are also extremely strenuous and should not be attempted by someone who is out of shape or who has lower back problems.

Leg lifts   Leg lifts are performed by lying flat on one's back and raising the legs about 6 to 12 inches off the floor for several seconds. One variation is to place the hands under the buttocks while lifting the legs. Another is to alternately pull the legs back toward the chest, making sure they remain off the floor when in the straightened position. Still another version is to do back-and-forth scissors kicks with the legs in the air.

Reverse back arches   Lie on the floor, facedown, then slowly lift both the legs and upper body off the floor. The weight of the body now rests on the front midsection and the pressure is most intense in the lower back. Hold the position for several seconds, then release and repeat. In addition, sets of twists and crunches, which are good for warm-ups, also make effective exercises during the workout.

Exercises for the Legs and the Cardiovascular System

With these exercises, as with others, common sense is essential for a safe and healthy workout. As previously mentioned, a beginner should choose a comfortable pace and then work up to more strenuous activity.

Chair and stair stepping   This is accomplished by standing in front of a chair or bench, stepping up onto the higher level, then stepping back down to the floor. There are two approaches to this exercise. The first is to do as many reps as possible in a given time period, perhaps two minutes. The number of reps completed will increase as a person's conditioning improves. The other approach is to do the reps at a slower pace for a longer time, perhaps 3 to 10 minutes, depending on the level of fitness.

A variation of this activity is to use the lowest stair or two of a staircase. A more difficult version is to climb the entire staircase repeatedly. This is very strenuous and should not be attempted during the first few weeks of exercise. In addition, despite the benefit it provides for the legs and cardiovascular system, stair climbing puts a great deal of pressure on the lower back. As a precaution, be careful to bend the knees and not to jolt the back while descending the stairs.

Running in place   Make sure to lift the legs at least 8 to 10 inches off the ground. A good strategy is to run in place at a moderate pace for a set time period, perhaps 5, 10, or 15 minutes, or to run as fast as possible for a shorter period.

Cycling   Using either a moving or stationary bike, novice cyclers should begin with a distance of about a half mile and work up to three miles or more. Comfortable, rhythmic breathing is essential.

Power walking   Power walking, also called *aerobic walking* or *fitness walking,* consists of walking at a very quick pace for several minutes. As with other aerobic activities, the longer the exercise lasts, the more beneficial it is. Power walks of 20, 30, or more minutes are best. Variations that increase the difficulty include swinging the arms vigorously in a rhythmic pattern and carrying small dumbbells while walking.

The jog-walk   This is perhaps the most strenuous beginner's exercise, and most people should attempt it only after several weeks of initial basic conditioning. After that, begin by power walking a certain distance, perhaps 100 yards, then run at a moderate pace for about the same distance. Continue to alternate running and walking over a total distance of at least a mile.

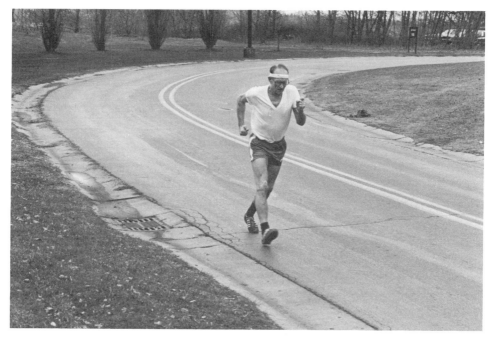

Power walks of at least 20 to 30 minutes provide a good aerobic workout.

MORE ADVANCED PROGRAMS

After a few months of basic conditioning, most people are ready for a more advanced exercise program. Since an advanced routine is much more strenuous than a beginner's workout, it is particularly essential to allow at least a day of rest for each major body area. A good strategy might be to work on upper body strength (using free weights or exercise machines) only once every two or three days and concentrate on strength training for the legs or abdominal muscles on the off days. If the program consists solely of one aerobic endurance exercise, such as jogging, cycling, swimming, rowing, power walking, or aerobic dance, a three-day-a-week schedule is usually best.

Programs that develop the upper body include weight lifting (with either free weights or exercise machines), rowing, and swimming.

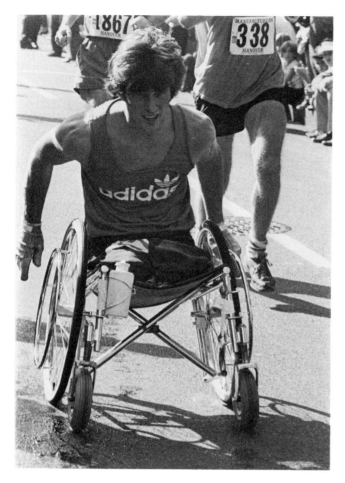

Physical handicaps need not inhibit an active life-style. The disabled can participate in sports ranging from skiing to swimming to track and field.

Rowing and swimming also develop cardiovascular endurance. Some programs for developing the lower body that are also excellent cardiovascular routines are running, cycling, power walking, and aerobic dancing.

Power walking, running, and cycling are performed the same way in an advanced program as they are in a beginning one. The difference is that distance and duration are increased. These factors will vary from individual to individual, but in general, a good rule of thumb is to make sure each aerobic workout lasts at least 45 minutes. Time permitting, an hour is even better. For the average person, this translates into a power walk of 3 to 5 miles, a run of 4 to 6 miles, or a bike ride of 9 to

12 miles. Trained athletes will be able to go even farther. Advanced aerobic dance workouts should also last 45 to 60 minutes. These can be done in formal classes with an instructor or exercise leader or at home.

Instructional books on aerobic dancing, running, walking, and cycling are available in the exercise or sports sections of most bookstores and libraries. After choosing an exercise discipline, it is a good idea to read up on the subject and consult people who have been practicing the routine for a long time. Also, for those who like the idea of combining fitness and social activities, many communities have exercise groups and clubs.

For those who prefer swimming, rowing, jogging on a track, riding a stationary bicycle, or lifting weights, advanced programs can be

Safe, effective exercise requires a combination of hard work, discipline, and common sense, but the rewards are a healthier body and a happier, more active life.

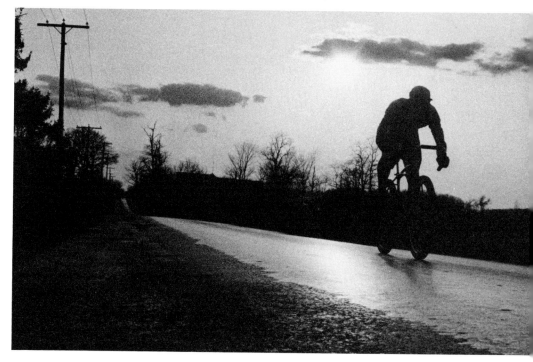

found at many health clubs and gyms, where expert advice from a coach or fitness instructor may also available. An individual planning to work out at home should look at instructional guides before beginning an advanced program. This is especially true for weight lifting, which is an excellent form of strength training but potentially dangerous if performed incorrectly.

Real physical fitness is not just a matter of working out a few times a week. Good and lasting health should be the goal of an ongoing life-style, a series of positive habits to be developed and maintained through life. A successful exercise program means combining sensible workouts with other good health habits, such as eating the proper foods; getting the right amount of sleep; and staying away from tobacco, alcohol, and drugs.

For some people, maintaining fitness is natural and easy. For many others, it is difficult, requiring constant reaffirmations of commitment and self-discipline. Yet those who are in good shape will testify that the rewards of fitness are well worth the effort to develop and maintain it. The benefits include a stronger, healthier body, fewer sick days, easier weight control, less fatigue, heightened feelings of pride and self-confidence, and a longer, happier life.

APPENDIX:
FOR MORE INFORMATION

The following is a list of organizations in the United States and Canada that can provide further information about exercise and related topics.

GENERAL INFORMATION

Aerobics and Fitness Association of
    America
15250 Ventura Blvd., Suite 310
Sherman Oaks, CA 91403
(818) 905-0040

American Aerobics Association
P.O. Box 401
Durango, CO 81301
(303) 247-4109

American College of Sports Medicine
P.O. Box 1440
Indianapolis, IN 46206-1440
(317) 637-9200

Canadian Association for Health, Physi-
    cal Education, and Recreation
1600 James Naismith Drive, Suite 606
Gloucester, Ontario
K1B 5N4
Canada
(613) 748-5622

Exercise Physiology Laboratory
University of Nevada at Las Vegas
School of Education

4505 Maryland Parkway
Las Vegas, NE 89154
(702) 739-3766

Exercise and Sports Research Institute
Rural Road
P.E.B.E Building
WYP-0404
Arizona State University
Tempe, AZ 85287
(602) 965-7510

IDEA (Association for Fitness Profes-
    sionals)
6190 Cornerstone Court E., Suite 204
San Diego, CA 92121-3773
(619) 535-8979

Institute for Aerobic Research
12330 Preston Road
Dallas, TX 75230
(214) 701-8001

Institute for Exercise Physiology and
    Health
University of Central Florida
College of Education
Department of Exceptional and Physical
    Education

Orlando, FL 32816
(407) 240-2049

President's Council on Physical Fitness
    and Sports
450 5th Street, NW, Suite 7103
Washington, DC 20001
(202) 272-3421

DIET AND NUTRITION

The American Dietetic Association
216 W. Jackson Blvd., Suite 800
Chicago, IL 60606-6995
(312) 899-0040

Food and Nutrition Information Center
National Agricultural Library
10301 Baltimore Blvd., Room 304
Beltsville, MD 20705
(301) 344-3719

National Institute of Nutrition
265 Carling Avenue, Suite 302
Ottawa, Ontario
K1S 2E1
Canada
(613) 235-3355

RUNNING

American Running and Fitness
    Association
9310 Old Georgetown Road
Bethesda, MD 20814
(301) 897-0197

Athletics Congress of the USA
200 S. Capitol Avenue, Suite 140
Indianapolis, IN 46225
(317) 261-0500

New York Road Runners Club
9 E. 89th Street
New York, NY 10128
(212) 860-4455

North American Network of Women
    Runners
P.O. Box 719
Bala Cynwyd, PA 19004
(215) 668-9886

YOGA

Ananda Marga
North American Headquarters
97-38 42nd Avenue
Corona, NY 11368
(718) 898-1603

Eureka Society
P.O. Box 1139
La Grange, TX 78945
(409) 968-3587

Himalayan International Institute of
    Yoga Science and Philosophy of
    the USA
R.R. 1, Box 400
Honesdale, PA 18431
(717) 253-5551

FURTHER READING

GENERAL INFORMATION

Barth, Christina. *Bodywork: Look Good—Keep Fit—Feel Great.* New York: Arco, 1987.

Bassey, E. J. *Exercise: The Facts.* New York: Oxford University Press, 1981.

Brown, Millie. *Low-Stress Fitness: The Low-Stress Way to Get in Shape.* Los Angeles: Price/Stern/Sloan, 1985.

Burke, Edmund J., ed. *Exercise, Science, and Fitness.* Longmeadow, MA: Mouvement, 1980.

Cantu, Robert C. *Exercise Injuries: Prevention and Treatment.* Washington, DC: Stone Wall Press, 1983.

Darden, Ellington. *Olympic Athletes Ask Questions About Exercise and Nutrition.* Ocoee, FL: Anna, N. d.

Davies, Bruce, and David Ashton. *Why Exercise?* New York: Blackwell, 1986.

Drews, Frederick R., et al. *A Healthy Life: Exercise, Behavior, Nutrition.* Indianapolis: Benchmark Press, 1986.

Hill, Grace. *Fitness First: Physical Exercises for All Ages.* Hanover, NH: Hill, 1980.

Jenner, Bruce, and Bill Dobbins. *Bruce Jenner's The Athletic Body: A Complete Fitness Guide for Teenagers.* New York: Simon & Schuster, 1984.

Katch, Frank I., and William D. McArdle. *Nutrition, Weight Control, and Exercise.* Philadelphia: Lea & Febiger, 1988.

Knight, Davis. *Flexibility: The Concept of Stretching and Exercise.* Dubuque: Kendall/Hunt, 1984.

Lewis, Sylvan R. *Diet and Exercise Made Easy.* Hollywood: Compact Books, 1980.

Liptak, Karen. *Aerobics Basics.* Englewood Cliffs, NJ: Prentice-Hall, 1983.

Manion, Jim, and Denie Manion. *Bodybuilding for Amateurs.* South Bend, IN: B & L, 1985.

Thomas, Gregory S., et al. *Exercise and Health: The Evidence and the Implications.* Boston: Oelgeschlager, 1981.

AEROBICS

Aerobics and Fitness Associations of America Staff. *Aerobics: Theory and Practice.* Costa Mesa, CA: HDL, 1987.

Klinger, A. K., et al. *The Complete Encyclopedia of Aerobics.* Longmeadow, MA: Mouvement, 1986.

Rosas, Debbie, et al. *Non-Impact Aerobics.* New York: Avon Books, 1988.

BODYBUILDING

McHugh, Thomas P. *Weight Training for Fitness and Sports.* Dubuque: Kendall/Hunt, 1984.

Schwarzenegger, Arnold, and Bill Dobbins. *Encyclopedia of Modern Bodybuilding*. New York: Simon and Schuster, 1987.

Sienna, Phillip A. *One Rep Max: A Guide to Beginning Weight Training Concepts and Principles*. Indianapolis: Benchmark Press, 1988.

Webster, David. *Body Building: An Illustrated History*. New York: Arco, 1982.

CALISTHENICS

Andrews, Keith, and Bruce J. Andrews. *Commuter Calisthenics: An Exercise Program for Busy People's Travel Time*. Evergreen, CO: Fitness Press, 1982.

Uram, Paul. *The Complete Stretching Book*. Mountain View, CA: Anderson World, 1980.

ISOMETRIC EXERCISE

Petrofsky, Jerold S. *Isometric Exercise and Its Clinical Implications*. Springfield, IL: Thomas, 1982.

Watson, Naomi. *Energize with Isometric Quickies*. Houston: Butterfly Press, 1977.

MARTIAL ARTS

Chow, David, and Richard Spangler. *Kung Fu, History, Philosophy, and Techniques*. Burbank: Unique, 1980.

Farkas, Emil, and John Corcoran. *Martial Arts: Traditions, History, People*. New York: W. H. Smith, 1980.

Hallander, Jane. *Complete Kung Fu Fighting Guide*. Burbank: Unique, 1985.

Queen, J. Allen. *Karate Handbook.* New York: Sterling, 1986.

Yeun, Kam. *Beginning Kung Fu.* Edited by Gilbert Johnson. Burbank: Ohara, 1975.

NUTRITION

Bosco, Dominick. *The People's Guide to Vitamins and Minerals: From A to Zinc.* Chicago: Contemporary Books, 1980.

Brooks, Svevo. *Common Sense Diet and Health.* Santa Cruz, CA: Botanica, 1987.

Carlson, Linda. *Food and Fitness.* Los Angeles: Price/Stern/Sloan, 1988.

Wade, Carlson. *Fact-Book on Fats, Oils, and Cholesterol.* New Canaan, CT: Keats, 1973.

RUNNING

Barley, Elizabeth G., and Mark Bloom. *Young Runner's Handbook.* New York: Warner Books, 1978.

Colfer, George R., and John M. Chevrette. *Running for Fun and Fitness: A Self-styled Program for Aerobic Running and Physical Fitness.* Dubuque: Kendall/Hunt, 1980.

Daws, Ron. *Running Your Best: The Committed Runner's Guide to Training and Racing.* East Rutherford, NJ: Stephen Greene Press, 1985

Dellinger, Bill, and Bill Freeman. *Competitive Runners Training Book.* New York: Macmillan, 1984.

Fixx, James F. *The Complete Book of Running.* New York: Random House, 1977.

Higdon, Hal. *Beginner's Running Guide.* Mountain View, CA: Anderson World, 1978.

Kostrubala, Thaddeus. *The Joy of Running.* New York: Pocket Books, 1986.

Valentine, Kim. *Teenage Distance Running.* Los Altos, CA: Tafnews, 1973.

YOGA

Ajaya, Swami. *Yoga Psychology: A Practical Guide to Meditation.* Honesdale, PA: Himalayan, 1976.

Bahadur, K. P. *The Wisdom of Yoga.* Livingston, NJ: Orient, 1977.

Kramer, Joel. *The Passionate Mind.* Berkeley: North Atlantic, 1983.

Udupa, K. N. *Stress and Its Management by Yoga.* Edited by R. C. Prasad. Columbia, MO: South Asia Books, 1986.

GLOSSARY

aerobic living, growing, or occurring only in the presence of oxygen

aerobics a system of exercises designed to improve cardiovascular fitness through increased oxygen consumption

alveoli tiny air sacs found in the lungs that allow oxygen to pass into the bloodstream

arteries tube-shaped vessels that carry blood away from the heart to various parts of the body

ascorbic acid vitamin C; a water-soluble vitamin found in many fruits and vegetables

atrophy a decrease in size or wasting away of an organ or tissue; muscles will atrophy from lack of use and lose their strength

blood pressure the pressure of blood on the walls of the arteries; it is usually recorded twice: once when the heart contracts and again when the heart is at rest

body composition the proportion of muscle to fat in various parts of the body; regular exercise can increase the ratio

bronchi air passages leading from the windpipe into the lungs

calisthenics a system of isotonic-type exercises or light gymnastics designed to maintain muscular strength

calories units based on the amount of heat or energy a food is capable of producing in the body; the more calories consumed, the more energy available; calories not used as energy are stored as fat; exercise burns calories, thus controlling body weight

capillaries tiny thin-walled blood vessels that allow oxygen to pass from the bloodstream into the tissues

carbohydrates a group of organic compounds, including sugars, starches, and celluloses, composed of carbon, hydrogen, and oxygen and generally produced by green plants; one of the three basic types of food

cardiac output the volume of blood pumped per minute from the left or right ventricle of the heart

cardiovascular system the system comprising the heart, the blood, and the blood vessels

cholesterol a pearly, waxlike substance found in all animal products, including meat, fats and oils, milk, and eggs

chronic fatigue the constant state of being tired and sluggish because of a consistent loss of sleep

circadian rhythm an organism's built-in daily patterns, apparently related to a variety of rhythms in the environment, including the cycles of day and night

connective tissue the strong tissue that holds together the bundles and fibers composing muscles

diaphragm a basin-shaped wall of muscle in the lower chest area that controls breathing, contracting and flattening with each inspiration (inhalation) and relaxing with each expiration (exhalation)

dyspnea difficult, labored breathing; normal when a result of vigorous work or athletic activity

emphysema a type of lung disease characterized by scarring of lung tissue, labored breathing, and a husky cough

eye-muscle coordination the brain's ability to guide the muscles and other body parts based on the images it receives from the eyes

fatigue weariness or exhaustion

fats compounds of carbon, hydrogen, and oxygen made from glycerol and fatty acid; the main substance into which excess carbohydrates are converted for storage by the body; one of the three basic types of food

fibers the threadlike structures that compose the muscles

hallucinogen a drug that provokes changes of sensation, thinking, self-awareness, and emotion

heart rate a measure of cardiac activity attained by monitoring the number of heartbeats per minute

hydrocarbons a compound made up of only carbon and hydrogen

ideal weight the healthiest weight for a particular height

inorganic compound a chemical compound that does not contain carbon

insomnia an inability to fall asleep or stay asleep

isometric contraction a contraction that occurs when a muscle tightens but is unable to move; often happens during an attempt to lift a heavy object that will not budge

isometric exercises exercises in which a muscle comes up against too much resistance to allow movement

isotonic contraction a contraction that enables a body part to move and, in turn, move an object

isotonic exercises exercises involving the contraction of a muscle, allowing for movement

kung fu a Chinese art of self-defense similar to karate

lactic acid an acid found in the blood; strenuous exercise can cause a buildup of lactic acid, resulting in muscle fatigue

ligaments fibrous bands of tissue that connect one bone to another in the region of a joint

minerals inorganic substances that carry out a variety of functions, including helping the body build bones, maintain cell structure, burn fuel, and transport oxygen through the bloodstream; to function properly, muscles must be constantly nourished by body fluids containing the correct proportion of minerals such as sodium, potassium, and calcium

minute volume of ventilation the amount of air breathed in and out per minute

muscular endurance the ability of a muscle to contract repeatedly

organic compound a chemical compound that contains carbon

proteins complex molecules consisting of a combination of amino acids; one of the three basic types of food

reaction time the amount of time it takes to respond to a given stimulus; if a person's reaction time is fast, he or she is said to have quick reflexes

respiratory system the body system that delivers oxygen to the lungs, the bloodstream, and the tissues and removes carbon dioxide

resting rate the heart rate when the body is at rest

resting value the volume of blood pumped by the heart per minute when the body is at rest

scurvy a disease caused by vitamin C deficiency; characterized by bleeding gums, loose teeth, and the slow healing of wounds

second wind the sudden feeling of relief and renewed ability to continue exercise following a period of labored breathing during a workout

steroids anabolic steroids; drugs similar to the male hormone testosterone that can increase muscle mass

stimulant any substance that increases, or speeds up, body functions

tendons tissues that connect muscles to bones

testosterone the male hormone responsible for inducing and maintaining male secondary sex characteristics, such as a deep voice and facial hair

tonus muscle tone; the tension or firmness of muscles

trachea the body's main air tube

veins vessels that carry blood from various parts of the body back to the heart

vitamins organic substances necessary for proper body function and essential to the nutrition of most animals and some plants

yoga a system of exercises designed to attain physical or mental control and well-being; introduced in ancient India and practiced by the Hindu priests as a means to clear the mind for prayer

INDEX

Acetyl coenzyme A, 68
Ada, Oklahoma, 77
Aerobic exercise, 53–54, 92, 93
Aerobics, 21, 49, 53
Alveoli, 45
Amateur Athletic Union (AAU), 28
Anaerobic exercise, 54
Arteries, 39. See also *Cardiovascular* system
Ascorbic acid, 69
Athens, 17
Atlas, Charles. *See* Siciliano, Andrew
Atrophy, 26

Baseball, 21, 55, 56, 57
Basedow, Johann, 20
Basketball, 21, 54
Beck, Charles, 21
Bicep, 26
Blood pressure, 39, 44. See also *Cardiovascular* system
Bodybuilding, 28–29, 33
Body composition, 34
Bone structure, 60
Boxing, 21, 58
Bronchi, 45

Calcium, 69, 70, 71
Calisthenics, 52–53

Calories, 62–67, 68. *See also* Exercise: and nutrition
Capillaries, 39
Carbohydrates, 67–68, 69
Carbon monoxide, 76
Cardiac output, 36, 37, 41
Cardiovascular system, 35–37, 38–39, 41, 44, 51, 54, 77, 79, 80, 82, 91
Center of gravity, 56
Central Florida, University of, 22
Central nervous system, 58
Chloride, 69
Cholesterol, 62, 71–72. *See also* Exercise: and nutrition
Chronic fatigue, 74
Circadian rhythm, 74
Citric acid, 68
Copper, 69
Crack, 79
Cross-country skiing, 54
Cycling, 92, 93, 94

Denmark, 19
Diaphragm, 23, 45. See also *Respiratory* system
Diastolic pressure, 41
Dyspnea, 45–46

Egypt, 16

Emphysema, 76
Encyclopedia of Bodybuilding (Schwarz-
    enegger), 29
Endurance, 31, 51, 53, 94
Exercise
    advanced programs, 93–96
    and alcohol use, 73, 78
    in ancient Egypt, 16
    in ancient Greece, 17–18
    in ancient Rome, 18
    approach for beginners, 60, 82–89
    balance, 58–60
    and cardiovascular system, 36–37, 39,
        41, 49, 91–92
    children, 14
    in China, 15
    and coordination, 57–58
    and drug use, 14, 73, 79
    and flexibility, 59–60, 82, 88
    and height, 55–56
    history, 14–20
    and injury, 86–87, 88
    and muscle use, 24, 26–27, 49
    and nutrition, 61–72
    and older people, 47–48
    and pain, 85
    and respiratory system, 44–47
    and sleep, 74–76
    and steroid use, 80
    and teenagers, 14
    and timing, 57–58
    and tobacco use, 14, 76–77
    in the United States, 20
    and warming up, 85, 88–89
    and weight, 13, 55, 64–65
Eye-muscle coordination, 55, 58

Fatigue, 30, 53, 82
Fats, 67–68, 69, 71–72. *See also* Exercise:
    and nutrition
Fibers, 24
Fixx, Jim, 62, 72
Follen, Charles, 21

Football, 56
Four basic food groups, 70

Germany, 19, 20
Glucose, 68
Glycogen, 30
Golf, 21
Great Britain, 19
Gymnastics, 55, 58, 59

Hallucinogens, 79. *See also* Exercise:
    and drug use
Handball, 54
Harvard step test, 42
Heart disease, 14, 47–48. See also *Car-
    diovascular* system
Heart rate, 37
Heatstroke, 86
Hepatitis, 75
Hinduism, 16
Hoboken, New Jersey, 21
Hydrocarbons, 76

Ice skating, 54, 58
Ideal weight, 55, 63. *See also* Exercise:
    and weight
India, 16
Inner ear, 59
Insomnia, 74, 79. *See also* Exercise: and
    sleep
Iodine, 69
Iron, 69
Isometric contractions, 27
Isometric exercise, 50–51, 90
Isotonic contractions, 27
Isotonic exercise, 51–52

Jahn, Friedrich Ludwig, 20, 21
Jahn societies, 20
Jennings, Herbert S., 14

Kong fu, 15
Krebs cycle, 68

Lactic acid, 30
Ligaments, 53, 60, 88

MacFadden, Bermarr, 28
Magnesium, 69
Malnutrition, 67
Marijuana, 79, 80. *See also* Exercise: and drug use
Marsee, Sean, 77
Massachusetts, 21
Middle Ages, 18, 19
Minerals, 18, 69
Minute volume of ventilation, 45
Mononucleosis, 75
Muscle contraction, 26
Muscle mass, 56–57
Muscle tone, 24
Muscular physique, 32, 33
Muths, Johann Christoph, 20

New York City, 28
Nicotine, 76, 77. *See also* Exercise: and tobacco use

Olympia, Greece, 18
Olympics, 18, 31. *See also* Exercise: and ancient Greece
Oral cancer, 77
Overload, 32
Oxaloacetic acid, 68

Park, Reg, 28. *See also* Bodybuilding
Pearl, Bill, 28
Phosphorus, 69
Plato, 14
Pneumonia, 75
Potassium, 69
Power walking, 54, 92, 93, 94
Proteins, 67–68, 69, 70. *See also* Exercise: and nutrition
Pumping Iron, 29
Push-ups, 89

Racquetball, 54
Radial artery, 42
Reaction time, 58
Reeves, Steve, 28
Respiratory system, 35, 44–46, 79, 84
Resting rate, 39
Resting value, 37
Rohter, Frank D., 22
Rome, 18
Rowing, 90, 93, 94, 95
Running, 58, 94

St. Louis, Missouri, 21
Sandow, Eugene, 28
Schwarzenegger, Arnold, 29, 32. *See also* Bodybuilding
Second wind, 46
Shin splints, 87
Siciliano, Andrew, 28
Sit-ups, 90
Skeletal muscles, 24, 47
Skiing, 21
Soccer, 54
Sodium, 69
Sphygmomanometer, 39
Spiess, Adolph, 20
Squash, 21, 54
Steroids, 29, 80
Stretching, 88
Sulfur, 69
Swimming, 21, 59, 93, 94, 95
Systolic pressure, 39

Tendons, 24
Tennis, 21, 57
Testosterone, 80
Tobacco, 73, 76–77, 80, 96
Tonus, 24
Trachea, 44
Track, 21
Training effect, 54

United States, 20

Vegetarianism, 70, 71. *See also* Exercise: and nutrition.
Veins, 39. See also *Cardiovascular* system
Vitamin A, 68
Vitamin C, 68
Vitamins, 68–69. *See also* Exercise: and nutrition

Warm-up, 30
Weight lifting, 93, 95, 96. *See also* Bodybuilding
Wrestling, 21, 56, 58

Yoga, 16

Zane, Frank, 28
Zinc, 69

PICTURE CREDITS

Alinari/Art Resource, NY: p. 15; Courtesy of American Cancer Society: p. 77; © American Running and Fitness Association: pp. 49, 83, 90, 95; © American Running and Fitness Association/Greg Merhar: pp. 31, 50, 52, 85, 91; American Running and Fitness Association/Redrawn by Gary Tong: p. 64; AP/Wide World Photos: pp. 70, 76, 79, 80; Art Resource, NY: p. 69; Marion Bernstein/Art Resource, NY: p. 13; The Bettmann Archive: pp. 19, 20, 21, 66, 74, 89; A. Castaigne/The Bettmann Archive: p. 17; Ann Chwatsky/Art Resource, NY: pp. 35, 94; Jan Lukas/Art Resource, NY: p. 56; Original illustrations by Robert Margulies: pp. 25, 38, 40, 46; Courtesy of National Heart, Lung, and Blood Institute/National Institutes of Health: p. 71; Original illustration by Nisa Rauschenberg: p. 63; Reuters/Bettmann Archive: pp. 34, 57, 59, 73; Rudolph R. Robinson/Art Resource, NY: pp. 41 (top), 75; Susan Rosenberg/Photo Researchers, Inc.: p. 78; © Pete Saloutos/The Stock Market: p. 43; Roger B. Smith/Art Resource, NY: p. 93; The Stock Market/Howard Sochurek, 1984: cover; Original illustrations by Gary Tong: pp. 26, 27, 36; United States Department of Agriculture: p. 67; UPI/Bettmann Archive: pp. 29, 30, 33, 53, 54, 61, 81; Vesalius/The Bettmann Archive: p. 23

Don Nardo is a writer, actor, filmmaker, and composer. He has written articles, short stories, and 15 books, as well as screenplays and teleplays, including work for Warner Bros. and ABC television. He has appeared in dozens of stage productions and has worked in front of or behind the camera in more than 20 films. His musical compositions, such as his oratorio *Richard III* and his film score for a version of *The Time Machine,* have been played by regional orchestras. An avid runner, wrestler, and fitness advocate, Mr. Nardo lives with his wife on Cape Cod, Massachusetts.

Dale C. Garell, M.D., is medical director of California Children Services, Department of Health Services, County of Los Angeles. He is also associate dean for curriculum at the University of Southern California School of Medicine and clinical professor in the Department of Pediatrics & Family Medicine at the University of Southern California School of Medicine. From 1963 to 1974, he was medical director of the Division of Adolescent Medicine at Children's Hospital in Los Angeles. Dr. Garell has served as president of the Society for Adolescent Medicine, chairman of the youth committee of the American Academy of Pediatrics, and as a forum member of the White House Conference on Children (1970) and White House Conference on Youth (1971). He has also been a member of the editorial board of the *American Journal of Diseases of Children.*

C. Everett Koop, M.D., Sc.D., is former Surgeon General, deputy assistant secretary for health, and director of the Office of International Health of the U.S. Public Health Service. A pediatric surgeon with an international reputation, he was previously surgeon-in-chief of Children's Hospital of Philadelphia and professor of pediatric surgery and pediatrics at the University of Pennsylvania. Dr. Koop is the author of more than 175 articles and books on the practice of medicine. He has served as surgery editor of the *Journal of Clinical Pediatrics* and editor-in-chief of the *Journal of Pediatric Surgery*. Dr. Koop has received nine honorary degrees and numerous other awards, including the Denis Brown Gold Medal of the British Association of Paediatric Surgeons, the William E. Ladd Gold Medal of the American Academy of Pediatrics, and the Copernicus Medal of the Surgical Society of Poland. He is a chevalier of the French Legion of Honor and a member of the Royal College of Surgeons, London.